T0326321

Curbside Consultation
in Pediatric Obesity

49 Clinical Questions

Curbside Consultation in Pediatrics
SERIES

SERIES EDITOR, LISA B. ZAOUTIS

Curbside Consultation
in Pediatric Obesity
49 Clinical Questions

EDITOR

Jeannie S. Huang, MD, MPH
University of California San Diego
Rady Children's Hospital
San Diego, California

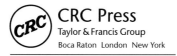

CRC Press
Taylor & Francis Group
Boca Raton London New York

CRC Press is an imprint of the
Taylor & Francis Group, an **informa** business

First published 2014 by SLACK Incorporated

Published 2024 by CRC Press
2385 NW Executive Center Drive, Suite 320, Boca Raton FL 33431

and by CRC Press
4 Park Square, Milton Park, Abingdon, Oxon, OX14 4RN

CRC Press is an imprint of Taylor & Francis Group, LLC

Library of Congress Cataloging-in-Publication Data

Curbside consultation in pediatric obesity : 49 clinical questions / editor, Jeannie S. Huang.
     p. ; cm. -- (Curbside consultation in pediatrics series)
  Includes bibliographical references and index.
  ISBN 978-1-61711-612-4 (paperback)
  I. Huang, Jeannie, editor of compilation. II. Series: Curbside consultation in pediatrics series.
  [DNLM: 1. Obesity. 2. Child. 3. Infant. 4. Pediatrics--methods. WD 210]
  RJ206
  618.92'398--dc23
                            2013044793

ISBN: 9781617116124 (pbk)
ISBN: 9781003523666 (ebk)

DOI: 10.1201/9781003523666

Dedication

I would like to dedicate this book to my parents, Song and Ann Huang, for giving me the foundation upon which to build a life and career; to my husband, Nat Chuang, for his constant support and love; to my three sons, Ethan, Jonah, and Benjamin, for giving me purpose for everything that I do; and finally, to my patients and families for challenging me as a clinician to address the things that matter and to improve my practice of medicine every day.

Contents

Acknowledgments

I would like to thank Dr. Lisa Zaoutis for giving me the opportunity to edit this book and to the many coauthors who have generously given their time and effort to make this book a reality. I also would like to recognize Carrie Kotlar of SLACK Incorporated for her help at every phase of development.

About the Editor

Jeannie S. Huang, MD, MPH obtained her BS from Brown University in Providence, RI and received her medical degree from the Johns Hopkins School of Medicine in Baltimore, MD. Her postdoctoral training included a pediatric residency at the Children's Hospital of Los Angeles in California and fellowship in the Combined Program in pediatric gastroenterology and nutrition at Boston Children's Hospital and Massachusetts General Hospital. She obtained a Master's of Public Health at the Harvard University School of Public Health, Boston, MA, in Clinical Effectiveness. She is currently Program Director of the Pediatric Gastroenterology, Hepatology and Nutrition fellowship program at the University of California San Diego (UCSD) and an associate professor of Pediatrics at UCSD. She is an active member of the North American Society of Pediatric Gastroenterology, Hepatology and Nutrition (NASPGHAN); she previously chaired the NASPGHAN Task Force on Obesity and currently leads quality improvement projects providing maintenance of certification credit in obesity as well as pediatric gastroenterology for both NASPGHAN and the American Academy of Pediatrics. Active in patient-oriented research, her main areas of interest are wide ranging but have primarily addressed how technology can be used to improve patient care and outcomes. She is the author of book chapters, review articles, and peer-reviewed manuscripts addressing pediatric obesity, among other topics related to pediatric care.

Contributing Authors

Richard L. Atkinson, MD (Question 10)
Clinical Professor of Pathology
Virginia Commonwealth University
Director, Obetech Obesity Research Center
Richmond, Virginia

Frank M. Biro, MD (Question 28)
Division of Adolescent and Transition Medicine
Cincinnati Children's Hospital Medical Center
Cincinnati, Ohio

Christopher F. Bolling, MD, FAAP (Question 35)
Pediatric Associates PSC
Crestview Hills, Kentucky
Obesity Chair, Kentucky Chapter of the
    American Academy of Pediatrics
Education Chair, Section on Obesity
American Academy of Pediatrics
Volunteer Associate Professor of Pediatrics
University of Cincinnati College of Medicine
Cincinnati, Ohio

Kerri N. Boutelle, PhD (Questions 38, 44)
Professor of Pediatrics and Psychiatry
University of California San Diego
La Jolla, California

Abby L. Braden, PhD (Questions 6, 33)
Department of Pediatrics
University of California San Diego
La Jolla, California

Lillian J. Choi, MD (Question 16)
Assistant Clinical Professor
Director of Endoscopy
Division of Pediatric Gastroenterology and
    Nutrition
University of California San Diego
Rady Children's Hospital
San Diego, California

Alison M. Coates, PhD (Question 27)
Nutritional Physiology Research Centre
Samsom Institute for Health Research
School of Health Sciences
University of South Australia
Adelaide, South Australia

Lee Ann E. Conard, RPh, DO, MPH (Question
    28)
Division of Adolescent and Transition Medicine
Cincinnati Children's Hospital Medical Center
Cincinnati, Ohio

Ellen L. Connor, MD (Question 20)
Associate Professor
Department of Pediatrics
Clinical Science Center
University of Wisconsin School of Medicine
    and Public Health
Madison, Wisconsin

Brian Dauenhauer, MEd (Question 12)
Assistant Professor
The University of Northern Colorado
School of Sport and Exercise Science
Greeley, Colorado

Christopher Davis, MD, PhD (Question 21)
University of California San Diego
Rady Children's Hospital
San Diego, California

Angela Estampador, BS, MPH (Question 22)
Department of Clinical Science
Genetic & Molecular Epidemiology Unit
Lund University
Malmö, Sweden

Katherine M. Flegal, PhD (Questions 2, 3)
Senior Research Scientist/Distinguished
    Consultant
National Center for Health Statistics
Centers for Disease Control and Prevention
Hyattsville, Maryland

Andrei Fodoreanu, MD (Question 18)
Department of Pediatrics
University of California San Diego
Rady Children's Hospital
San Diego, California

Paul W. Franks, Bsc(Hons), MS, MPhil (Cantab), PhD (Cantab), FTOS (Question 22)
Head of Genetic & Molecular Epidemiology Unit
Department of Clinical Science
Lund University
Malmö, Sweden
Adjunct Professor of Nutrition
Harvard School of Public Health
Boston, Massachusetts
Professor of Molecular Epidemiology
Department of Public Health & Clinical Medicine
Umeå University
Umeå, Sweden

Jeanette M. Garcia, MS (Question 37)
Kinesiology Program
Curry School of Education
University of Virginia
Charlottesville, Virginia

Mary Abigail S. Garcia, MD (Question 15)
Department of Pediatrics
Division of Pediatric Gastroenterology, Hepatology and Nutrition
University of California San Diego
Rady Children's Hospital
San Diego, California

Dara Garner-Edwards, MSW, LCSW (Question 26)
Department of Pediatrics
Wake Forest School of Medicine
Brenner FIT Program
Brenner Children's Hospital
Winston-Salem, North Carolina

Michael Gottschalk, MD, PhD (Question 18)
Clinical Professor of Pediatrics
Vice Chair Education
Chief, Pediatric Endocrinology
University of California San Diego
Rady Children's Hospital
San Diego, California

David Gozal, MD (Question 8)
The Herbert T. Abelson Professor and Chair
Department of Pediatrics
Pritzker School of Medicine
Physician-in-Chief, Comer Children's Hospital
The University of Chicago
Chicago, Illinois

H. Mollie Grow, MD, MPH (Question 29)
Assistant Professor, General Pediatrics
Seattle Children's Hospital
University of Washington
Seattle, Washington

Rohit Gupta, MD, PhD (Questions 31, 47)
Fellow
Pediatric Gastroenterology and Hepatology
Seattle Children's Hospital
University of Washington
School of Medicine
Seattle, Washington

Sarah Hampl, MD (Question 30)
Medical Director, Weight Management
Children's Mercy Hospitals and Clinics
Associate Professor of Pediatrics
University of Missouri-Kansas City
School of Medicine
Kansas City, Missouri

Sandra Hassink, MD, FAAP (Questions 32, 39)
Director Nemours Obesity Initiative
Division of Weight Management
Nemours/Alfred I. duPont Hospital for Children
Wilmington, Delaware

Kimberly Henrichs, MD (Question 20)
Fellow
Department of Pediatrics
Clinical Science Center
University of Wisconsin School of Medicine
    and Public Health
Madison, Wisconsin

Krista Beth Highland, PhD (Question 23)
Cancer Prevention & Control Program
Lombardi Comprehensive Cancer Center
Georgetown University Medical Center
Washington, DC

Linda L. Hill, MD, MPH (Question 43)
Professor
Director of Preventive Medicine Residency
Department of Family and Preventive Medicine
University of California San Diego
La Jolla, California

Stefanie N. Hinkle, PhD (Question 7)
Postdoctoral Fellow
Division of Intramural Population Health
    Research
Eunice Kennedy Shriver National Institute of
    Child Health and Human Development
National Institutes of Health
Bethesda, Maryland

Nancy Hoo, MD (Question 1)
University of California San Diego
Rady Children's Hospital
San Diego, California

Sherry Huang, MD (Question 1)
University of California San Diego
Rady Children's Hospital
San Diego, California

Xiaofen Deng Keating, PhD (Questions 11, 13, 14)
Associate Professor
Department of Curriculum and Instruction
The University of Texas at Austin
Austin, Texas

Jacqueline Kerr, PhD (Question 9)
Center for Wireless & Population Health
    Systems
Department of Family and Preventive Medicine
University of California San Diego
La Jolla, California

Brian K. Kit, MD, MPH (Questions 2, 3)
Medical Officer
National Center for Health Statistics
Centers for Disease Control and Prevention
Hyattsville, Maryland

Stephanie Knatz, PhD (Questions 38, 44)
Postdoctoral Fellow
Department of Pediatrics and Psychiatry
University of California San Diego
La Jolla, California

Heather M. Kong, MD (Questions 19, 24)
Rutgers
New Jersey Medical School
Newark, New Jersey

Kirsten La, PharmD, BCPS (Question 46)
Pharmacist Clinical Specialist
Long Beach Memorial Medical Center and
    Miller Children's Hospital Long Beach
Long Beach, California

*Jennifer Le, PharmD, MAS, BCPS-ID, FCCP,
    FCSHP (Questions 41, 46)*
Associate Professor of Clinical Pharmacy
University of California San Diego
Skaggs School of Pharmacy and Pharmaceutical
    Sciences
La Jolla, California

Colleen Taylor Lukens, PhD (Question 45)
Pediatric Psychologist
Department of Child and Adolescent Psychiatry
    and Behavioral Sciences
The Children's Hospital of Philadelphia
Philadelphia, Pennsylvania

Kimberly Montez, MD (Question 16)
Adolescent and Pediatric Medicine Unit
Massachusetts General Hospital for Children
MGH Chelsea HealthCare Center
Chelsea, Massachusetts

Tamasyn Nelson, DO (Question 48)
Department of Pediatrics
Bellevue Hospital Center
New York, New York

Kimberly P. Newton, MD (Questions 17, 40)
Assistant Professor
Department of Pediatrics
Division of Pediatric Gastroenterology,
    Hepatology and Nutrition
Interim Medical Director of Pediatric Liver
    Transplant
Director of the Pediatric Celiac Disease Clinic
University of California San Diego
Rady Children's Hospital
San Diego, California

Kevin Patrick, MD, MS (Question 36)
Professor, Family and Preventive Medicine
Director, Center for Wireless and Population
    Health Systems
The Qualcomm Institute of Calit2
University of California San Diego
La Jolla, California

Denise Purdie, MD (Question 15)
Department of Pediatrics
University of California San Diego
Rady Children's Hospital
San Diego, California

Kyung E. Rhee, MD, MSc, MA (Questions 6, 33)
Assistant Professor of Pediatrics
Department of Pediatrics
Center for Community Health
University of California San Diego
La Jolla, California

Sanjeev Sabharwal, MD, MPH (Questions 19, 24)
Professor, Department of Orthopaedics
Chief, Pediatric Orthopaedics
Rutgers—New Jersey Medical School
Newark, New Jersey

Jeffrey B. Schwimmer, MD (Question 17)
Professor of Pediatrics
Division of Gastroenterology, Hepatology, and
    Nutrition
Department of Pediatrics
Director of the Fatty Liver Clinic
Department of Gastroenterology
University of California San Diego
Rady Children's Hospital
San Diego, California

Rulan Shangguan, PhD (Questions 11, 13, 14)
PhD Candidate, Graduate Assistant
Department of Curriculum and Instruction
The University of Texas at Austin
Austin, Texas

Andrea J. Sharma, PhD (Question 7)
Division of Reproductive Health
National Center for Chronic Disease Prevention
    and Health Promotion
Centers for Disease Control and Prevention
Atlanta, Georgia
US Public Health Service Commissioned Corps
Atlanta, Georgia

John R. Sirard, PhD (Question 37)
Kinesiology Department and Youth-Nex
    Research Center
Curry School of Education
University of Virginia
Charlottesville, Virginia

Joseph A. Skelton, MD, MS (Question 26)
Department of Pediatrics
Wake Forest School of Medicine
Brenner FIT Program
Brenner Children's Hospital
Winston-Salem, North Carolina

Karen Stephens, MS, RD, CSP, LD (Question 30)
Manager, Nutrition and Lactation Services
PHIT Kids Dietitian
Children's Mercy Hospitals and Clinics
Kansas City, Missouri

David L. Suskind, MD (Questions 31, 17)
Associate Professor of Pediatrics
Division of Gastroenterology, Hepatology and
    Nutrition
Seattle Children's Hospital
University of Washington
Seattle, Washington

Kenneth P. Tercyak, PhD (Question 23)
Cancer Prevention & Control Program
Lombardi Comprehensive Cancer Center
Georgetown University Medical Center
Washington, DC

Leonardo Trasande, MD, MPP (Question 48)
Associate Professor
Departments of Population Health,
    Environmental Medicine and Pediatrics
New York University Langone Medical Center
New York, New York

Patrika Tsai, MD (Questions 4, 5)
Pediatric Gastroenterologist
University of California San Francisco
Benioff Children's Hospital
San Francisco, California

Raymond J. Tseng, DDS, PhD (Question 25)
Department of Pediatric Dentistry
University of North Carolina
Chapel Hill, North Carolina
Department of Public Health
Campbell University College of Pharmacy &
    Health Sciences
Buies Creek, North Carolina
High House Pediatric Dentistry
Cary, North Carolina

Margarita D. Tsiros, PhD (Question 27)
Lecturer in Health Sciences (Physiotherapy)
Nutritional Physiology Research Centre
Samsom Institute for Health Research
School of Health Sciences
University of South Australia
Adelaide, South Australia

Victor E. Uko, MD, MRCPCH (UK) (Question 40)
Pediatric Gastroenterologist
Department of Pediatric Specialties
Gundersen Health Systems
La Crosse, Wisconsin

Christine Wood, MD, FAAP, CLE (Question 49)
Co-Chair, San Diego County Childhood
    Obesity Initiative
El Camino Pediatrics
Encinitas, California

Stavra A. Xanthakos, MD, MS (Questions 34, 42)
Medical Director
Surgical Weight Loss Program for Teens
Co-Director, Steatohepatitis Center
Associate Professor of Pediatrics
Division of Gastroenterology, Hepatology and
    Nutrition
Cincinnati Children's Hospital Medical Center
Cincinnati, Ohio

Introduction

The role of the clinician in the management of obesity is a challenging one. One has to balance prevention with accurate assessment and treatment of associated comorbidities along with appropriate counseling for the family at risk. To accomplish this within the limited time afforded to the general practitioner at an outpatient visit is unrealistic and yet expected.

In the following 49 chapters, practical and challenging questions alike are addressed in detail and coupled with useful and practical advice for the busy clinician. The book as a whole strongly endorses the multidisciplinary approach to the care of the patient with weight-related issues. As such, chapters are written by a wide variety of health care practitioners, public health advocates, and researchers. These select experts in their respective fields provide valuable perspective and demonstrate how integrating care from professionals from multiple health fields can result in better and best outcomes for children and families dealing with overweight and obesity.

I am of course indebted to my many coauthors for their contributions to this book. Their brief but impactful responses will provide the relevant clinical pearls for the general practitioner to integrate into his or her clinical practices in weight management and obesity prevention. I hope that you will find this book to be relevant, practical, and helpful to your practice of medicine.

Jeannie S. Huang, MD, MPH

SECTION I

EPIDEMIOLOGY

OBESITY IN CHILDREN SEEMS TO BE COMMON. IS THIS AN EPIDEMIC? IS THIS TRUE OUTSIDE OF THE UNITED STATES?

Sherry Huang, MD and Nancy Hoo, MD

Obesity among children and adolescents has become a public health crisis. In the United States (US), overweight and obesity are determined by the body mass index (BMI) for each age-gender group. As defined by the Centers for Disease Control and Prevention, children aged 2 years and older with a BMI between the 85th and 95th percentile are overweight, and those with a BMI greater than the 95th percentile are obese. Children with a BMI greater than the 97th percentile are severely obese. As of 2010, 16.9% of US children and adolescents aged 2 to 19 years were obese and 31.8% were either obese or overweight.[1] There are significant differences in obesity prevalence based on sex, age, and socioeconomic status. Racial differences also exist but will be discussed separately in Question 3. The prevalence of obesity is higher among male children and adolescents (18.6%) compared with female children and adolescents (16%). Adolescents also have a higher prevalence of obesity compared with preschool-aged children. Obesity disproportionately affects children from low socioeconomic backgrounds, affecting 1 in 7 preschool-aged children of low income.[1]

In the past 3 decades, the prevalence of obesity in the US has increased dramatically among all age groups. Between the 1970s and 2008, obesity rates among children nearly tripled in all age groups (ages 2 to 5 years from 5% to 15.4%; ages 6 to 11 years from 6.5% to 19.6%; and ages 12 to 19 years from 5% to 18.1%).[1] Obesity trends have varied by sex, age, race and ethnicity, and socio-economic status. During the 12 years between 1999 and 2010, the prevalence of obesity increased in male children and adolescents, but remained unchanged in female children and adolescents.[1] Although BMI trends among African American and White children aged 6 to 11 years have increased over this time frame, African American children experienced a 5-fold increase in obesity prevalence compared with a 3-fold increase in White children.[2] Factors contributing to the rise in obesity include sedentary lifestyles and increased caloric intake of processed, calorie-rich foods.

Huang JS, ed. *Curbside Consultation in Pediatric Obesity: 49 Clinical Questions* (pp 3-4).
© 2014 Taylor & Francis Group

The epidemic trend in obesity has also been observed globally in developed and developing countries. However, comparison of obesity prevalence data between the US and other countries may be limited by the use of different classification systems. Between 2009 and 2010, the prevalence of overweight and obesity in preschool-aged children globally was 6.7%.[3] Over the past 2 decades, the prevalence of obesity has doubled in developed countries when compared with developing countries.[3] During this time, developing and developed countries have demonstrated an increase in the prevalence of overweight and obese preschool-aged children, with developing countries increasing at a higher proportion compared with developed countries.[3] As of 2006, the countries with the highest prevalence of overweight children included the US, Europe, and parts of the Western Pacific.[4] In the US and Europe (Great Britain, southern aspects of Western Europe-Greece, Italy, Malta, Spain, and Portugal), more than 15% of the youth are noted to be overweight. There is a notably lower obesity prevalence of 10% to 15% in Nordic European countries and the majority of countries in Eastern Europe.[5] The regional differences in overweight and obesity may be explained by a number of factors, including differences in socioeconomic status and the availability and preference of food and leisure-time physical activities.

Obesity in childhood has been associated with numerous medical and psychosocial comorbidities. (Comorbidities will be further addressed in Section V.) Overweight children and adolescents have a higher likelihood of developing dyslipidemia, elevated blood pressure, type 2 diabetes, and nonalcoholic fatty liver disease. Pulmonary disorders such as obstructive sleep apnea are observed more frequently in obese children. Orthopedic complications observed in higher association with pediatric obesity include Blount disease and slipped capital femoral epiphysis. The psychological consequences of childhood obesity include increased risky behaviors such as cigarette smoking in adolescence, increased likelihood as perpetrators and victims of bullying, and increased social marginalization. Paralleling the overall increase in obesity has been a rise in numerous childhood comorbidities and, subsequently, adult morbidity and mortality.

Children who have high BMIs are more likely to have high BMIs in adulthood. Children and adolescents with BMIs greater than the 95th percentile have a higher likelihood of being overweight at age 35 years, with greater correlation in older children. Obese adults who were obese as children have higher cardiovascular risks, including type 2 diabetes, dyslipidemia, hypertension, and carotid atherosclerosis, compared with those who were not obese as children. These associated cardiovascular risk factors increase adult mortality. However, cardiovascular risk does not appear limited to those meeting criteria for overweight and obesity. In fact, children with BMIs greater than the 75th percentile have twice the likelihood of mortality from ischemic heart disease compared with children with BMIs between the 25th and 48th percentile.

Childhood obesity is a global epidemic and health care crisis. Public health interventions aimed at addressing childhood overweight and obesity thus have the potential to reduce the significant burden of associated morbidity and mortality in childhood through adulthood.

References

1. Ogden C, Carroll M. Prevalence of obesity among children and adolescents: United States, trends 1963-1965 through 2007-2008. Cross-national comparison of childhood obesity: the epidemic and the relationship between obesity and socioeconomic status. Atlanta, GA: Centers for Disease Control and Prevention, National Center for Health Statistics; 2010.
2. Freedman DS, Khan LK, Serdula MK, Ogden CL, Dietz WH. Racial and ethnic differences in secular trends for childhood BMI, weight, and height. *Obesity (Silver Spring)*. 2012;14(2):301-308.
3. de Onis M, Blössner M, Borghi E. Global prevalence and trends of overweight and obesity among preschool children. *Am J Clin Nutr*. 2010;92(5):1257-1264.
4. Wang Y, Lobstein T. Worldwide trends in childhood overweight and obesity. *Int J Pediatr Obes*. 2006;1(1):11-25.
5. Janssen I, Katzmarzyk PT, Boyce WF, et al. Comparison of overweight and obesity prevalence in school-aged youth from 34 countries and their relationships with physical activity and dietary patterns. *Obes Rev*. 2005;6(2):123-132.

QUESTION

2

Obesity In Children Seems to Be Common. Are the Current Definitions of Obesity Accurate, and What Are They Based On?

Brian K. Kit, MD, MPH and Katherine M. Flegal, PhD

Disclaimer: The findings and conclusions in this report are those of the authors and not necessarily those of the Centers for Disease Control and Prevention (CDC).

Obesity is an excess of adiposity or body fat. Therefore, central to the definition of obesity is the determination of the level of adiposity that qualifies as "excess." This level has been broadly described as the point beyond which a child's health and well-being is negatively affected. Adiposity can be measured using various methods, including underwater weighing, measurements of skinfold thickness, bioelectrical impedance analysis, waist circumference measures, and radiologic imaging such as dual-energy X-ray absorptiometry. However, obtaining accurate measures of adiposity can be time consuming, expensive, and impractical in clinical practice. Moreover, no accepted standards exist to define the level of adiposity beyond which negative effects occur.

According to current definitions, approximately 17% of children and adolescents in the United States are obese.[1] This estimate is based on the most commonly used definition of obesity, which uses weight and height measures combined as body mass index (BMI; weight [kilograms]/height^2 [meters]).[2] Thus, BMI is calculated using weight and height and is not a measure of adiposity. By dividing weight by the square of height, BMI adjusts weight for height and allows for a comparison of weight independent of height. Among children, normal growth includes sex- and age-specific patterns of adipose tissue accumulation and BMI changes; therefore, the BMI of a child is generally assessed relative to the BMI of children of the same sex and age. Obesity is then defined by comparing a child's BMI to a reference population of children of the same sex and age using growth charts.

Growth charts have been widely used to monitor growth in children, but their use to identify children with obesity is a more recent example of their use in clinical medicine. Many growth charts are available, including those based on children from a specific country and those based on

Huang JS, ed. *Curbside Consultation in Pediatric Obesity: 49 Clinical Questions* (pp 5-6).
© 2014 Taylor & Francis Group

children from multiple countries. Two commonly used growth charts are the 2000 CDC growth charts, a growth reference for children and adolescents aged 0 to 19 years, and the 2006 World Health Organization growth charts, a growth standard for children aged 0 to 5 years.[3] A growth reference is based on data collected during a specific time period within a specific population and describes how children *did* grow. On the other hand, a growth standard is generally based on a highly selective sample of children who meet specific requirements (for example, breastfeeding norms, standard pediatric care, and nonsmoking) and describes how children *should* grow. Although different growth charts may use a different approach for sample selection, the statistical methods used to create the growth charts are generally similar.

Currently, the American Academy of Pediatrics and the US government define childhood obesity for children aged 2 years and above as a BMI greater than or equal to the sex- and age-specific 95th percentile of the 2000 CDC Growth Charts. These growth charts are based on nationally representative data from US children surveyed in the 1960s and 1970s and, among children aged 0 to 6 years, the late 1980s and early 1990s.[4] This definition of childhood obesity is statistically defined and not based on clinical outcomes. An explicit outcomes-based rationale for choosing a particular BMI cutoff point to define obesity has not been described. Nevertheless, current research demonstrates associations between current CDC Growth Chart–defined overweight and obesity states and adverse outcomes, as will be discussed in the subsequent chapters.

There are limitations to the use of BMI to define obesity. BMI is not a direct measure of adiposity, although it correlates well with measures of adiposity, and children with high BMIs tend to have high adiposity. However, lean body mass, including muscle and bone mass, contributes to a child's weight; therefore, a child with high lean body mass may also have a high BMI. In the clinical setting, there are no practical tools to distinguish high adiposity from high lean body mass; therefore, the American Academy of Pediatrics' Expert Committee recommends that clinicians consider factors other than a child's BMI percentile in the clinical evaluation of obesity, including family history of obesity and medical problems, the child's past BMI pattern, and the child's current medical conditions and current health behaviors.[2]

In the US, data from national health examination surveys show that approximately 17% of 2- to 19-year-olds were obese between 2009 and 2010, defined using the sex- and age-specific 95th BMI percentile of the 2000 CDC Growth Charts. The 17% obesity prevalence is an accurate estimate of childhood obesity in the US using established definitions based on BMI. However, obesity prevalence estimates will differ depending on the growth charts used. Regardless of the growth charts used, obesity prevalence estimates are based on a measure of body weight adjusted for height rather than on adiposity. Obesity prevalence estimates based on BMI may not accurately reflect the number of children and adolescents in the US with excess adiposity. Some children with excess adiposity may not be identified by use of the BMI based definition of obesity, and some children who are identified as obese by use of the BMI-based definition of obesity do not necessarily have excess adiposity.

References

1. Ogden CL, Carroll MD, Kit BK, Flegal KM. Prevalence of obesity and trends in body mass index among US children and adolescents, 1999-2010. *JAMA*. 2012;307(5):483-490.
2. Barlow SE; Expert Committee. Expert committee recommendations regarding the prevention, assessment, and treatment of child and adolescent overweight and obesity: summary report. *Pediatrics*. 2007;120(Suppl 4):S164-S192.
3. Grummer-Strawn LM, Reinold C, Krebs NF; Centers for Disease Control and Prevention. Use of World Health Organization and CDC growth charts for children aged 0-59 months in the United States. *MMWR Recomm Rep*. 2010;59(RR-9):1-15.
4. Kuczmarski RJ, Ogden CL, Guo SS, et al. 2000 CDC Growth Charts for the United States: methods and development. *Vital Health Stat 11*. 2002;246:1-190.

Obesity in Children Seems to Be More Common in Non-White Racial Groups. What Racial Groups Are at Particular Risk, and What Considerations Are Important for Each?

Brian K. Kit, MD, MPH and Katherine M. Flegal, PhD

Disclaimer: The findings and conclusions in this report are those of the authors and not necessarily those of the Centers for Disease Control and Prevention.

In the United States, 17% of children are obese, and race-ethnic differences in childhood obesity based on body mass index (BMI) have been well described.[1] Generally, based on data from the National Health and Nutrition Examination Surveys (NHANES), non-Hispanic Black and Hispanic children have a higher prevalence of obesity than non-Hispanic White children, whereas other research suggests Asian American children have a lower obesity prevalence than non-Hispanic White children. Within broadly defined race-ethnic groups, there may be variations in obesity prevalence. For example, in one study of 4 year olds, US children of Vietnamese ethnicity had a higher obesity prevalence than those of Asian Indian ethnicity.

Race-ethnic differences in childhood obesity prevalence, defined using BMI, may not reflect differences in adiposity. BMI, a measure of body weight adjusted for height, is correlated with other measures of adiposity but is a proxy measure, rather than a direct measure, of adiposity. Analyses using dual-energy x-ray absorptiometry, a more direct measure of adiposity, suggest that there are significant race-ethnic differences in adiposity that are not always consistent, and in some instances inconsistent, with race-ethnic differences in obesity, as measured by BMI.

In general, non-Hispanic Black boys have a lower percentage of body fat than non-Hispanic White boys, but non-Hispanic Black and White girls have similar percentages of body fat.[2] Thus, despite a significantly higher prevalence of obesity, as measured by BMI, among non-Hispanic Black children, this group does not have a higher percentage of body fat than non-Hispanic White children. Mexican American children have a higher prevalence of obesity, as measured by BMI,

Huang JS, ed. *Curbside Consultation in Pediatric Obesity: 49 Clinical Questions* (pp 7-9).

and a higher percentage of body fat than non-Hispanic White children. Data describing percentage of body fat among Asian-American children are more limited but Asian American adults tend to have lower BMIs but higher adiposity than non-Hispanic White adults.

Among boys and girls, at a given range of BMI percentiles, including the BMI percentile corresponding to the obesity cutoff point of ≥95th percentile, there are race-ethnic differences in percentage body fat. Generally, non-Hispanic Black children have a lower percentage of body fat at a given BMI value than do non-Hispanic White and Mexican American children. The difference between race-ethnic groups in percentages of body fat at specified BMI percentile cutoff points suggests the disparities in childhood obesity prevalence using BMI do not entirely reflect differences in adiposity. There are race-ethnic differences in lean body mass, including muscle and bone mass, that contribute to the differences between BMI and body fat classifications.

Often-cited concerns associated with childhood obesity include the tracking of childhood obesity into adulthood and the association between childhood obesity and markers of cardiovascular health, including elevated blood pressure, adverse lipid concentrations, and glucose intolerance.[3] Moreover, some markers of cardiovascular health, including hypertension, also track from childhood to adulthood. Understanding differences by race-ethnicity in tracking obesity and markers of cardiovascular health has been the focus of past research; reducing these disparities is of importance nationally.

Although there are differences among boys across race-ethnicity groups in obesity prevalence as measured by BMI, among adult men there are few differences in obesity prevalence between non-Hispanic White, non-Hispanic Black, and Hispanic men. Among girls, race-ethnic differences in obesity prevalence as measured by BMI begin in childhood and continue into adulthood. Few studies have specifically examined race-ethnic differences in obesity tracking.

Because childhood obesity is associated with adverse cardiovascular markers, it would be expected that groups with a higher obesity prevalence as measured by BMI would have more adverse cardiovascular risk factors. However, this has not been consistently shown for markers of cardiovascular health, including elevated blood pressure, adverse lipid concentrations, and glucose intolerance. For example, using data from NHANES, 3.1%, 3.2%, and 2.0% of non-Hispanic White, non-Hispanic Black, and Mexican American youth, respectively, have measured blood pressures consistent with hypertension. Likewise, high serum low-density lipoprotein cholesterol concentration is similar for non-Hispanic White (7.7%), non-Hispanic Black (8.9%), and Hispanic (5.4%) adolescents. Prevalence of low serum high-density lipoprotein cholesterol, which is more strongly correlated with obesity than low-density lipoprotein cholesterol, is lower among non-Hispanic Black adolescents (9.1%) than non-Hispanic White (15.3%) and Mexican American (17.7%) adolescents. The prevalence of impaired fasting glucose is significantly different across race-ethnic groups but not consistent with differences in obesity prevalence. Despite a higher obesity prevalence as measured by BMI among non-Hispanic Black adolescents, the prevalence of impaired fasting glucose is lower in this group than in non-Hispanic White adolescents. Similarities and differences in markers of cardiovascular health by race-ethnicity are consistent overall for boys and girls.

Obesity is one factor that contributes to abnormalities in markers of cardiovascular health. However, other factors, including family history, physical activity, dietary patterns, and tobacco use, contribute to adverse markers of cardiovascular health.[4] Differences in these factors, alone or in combination, may in part explain the similar, or in some cases lower, burden for markers of cardiovascular health despite a higher obesity prevalence among specific race-ethnic groups. Race-ethnic differences in percentage body fat at a given BMI may also contribute to this finding. Current clinical practice guidelines include recommendations for screening and early detection of obesity and markers of cardiovascular health.[3] These guidelines are applicable to youth of all race-ethnic groups. The Health Disparities and Inequalities Report-United States, 2011, from the Centers for Disease Control and Prevention suggests, among other measures, that educational efforts to promote healthy eating and active living may reduce race-ethnic disparities in obesity prevalence.

References

1. Ogden CL, Carroll MD, Kit BK, Flegal KM. Prevalence of obesity and trends in body mass index among US children and adolescents, 1999-2010. *JAMA*. 2012;307(5):483-490.
2. Flegal KM, Ogden CL, Yanovski JA, et al. High adiposity and high body mass index-for-age in US children and adolescents overall and by race-ethnic group. *Am J Clin Nutr*. 2010;91(4):1020-1026.
3. Barlow SE; Expert Committee. Expert committee recommendations regarding the prevention, assessment, and treatment of child and adolescent overweight and obesity: summary report. *Pediatrics*. 2007;120(Suppl 4):S164-S192.
4. Expert Panel on Integrated Guidelines for Cardiovascular Health Risk Reduction in Children Adolescents, National Heart Lung Blood Institute. Expert panel on integrated guidelines for cardiovascular health and risk reduction in children and adolescents: summary report. *Pediatrics*. 2011;128(Suppl 5):S213-S256.

SECTION II

PATHOPHYSIOLOGY/ DEVELOPMENT OF CHILDHOOD OBESITY

WHAT BODY SYSTEMS AFFECT THE DEVELOPMENT OF OBESITY?

Patrika Tsai, MD

Many body systems play a role in the development of obesity, either directly or indirectly. These systems include the nervous, musculoskeletal, respiratory, cardiovascular, immune, integumentary, reproductive, gastrointestinal, and endocrine systems. Problems with any of these systems may affect energy expenditure, caloric intake, and energy homeostasis, which can increase the risk for obesity. The development of obesity in various disease states highlights the contribution of each body system to weight maintenance.

Body systems that enable physical activity are important in energy expenditure. Patients with decreased mobility or activity secondary to underlying neuromuscular conditions like muscular dystrophy or cerebral palsy will have relatively low energy expenditure compared with those without such conditions. Similarly, pulmonary function is critical for exercise, and individuals with poorly controlled asthma may avoid physical activity because they have breathing difficulties while exercising and participating in sports. Those with obstructive sleep apnea often suffer from daytime fatigue, which affects motivation for activity. People with cardiac disease may have limitations on their ability to increase cardiac output, which then reduces the level of activity. Even the immune and integumentary systems can play a role indirectly. For example, although bone marrow transplant patients may be able to perform physical activity, they may be restricted from recreational activities in crowded areas owing to concern for infection given their immunodeficient state. Similarly, people are also now more aware of sun exposure as a risk factor for skin cancers, and current recommendations to avoid the sun during peak hours may limit time available for physical activity. Many body systems, therefore, play a part in energy expenditure.

Although it is easy to attribute obesity to simply eating too much or to excess caloric intake, the interactions between the brain, the gastrointestinal system, and the endocrine system to maintain energy homeostasis are extremely complex. Several hormones are involved in transmitting hunger and satiety signals, and dysregulation of these signals contributes to obesity. Ghrelin is the only

Huang JS, ed. *Curbside Consultation in*
Pediatric Obesity: 49 Clinical Questions (pp 13-15).
© 2014 Taylor & Francis Group

known orexigenic or appetite-stimulating gut hormone and is secreted mainly by the stomach. Ghrelin levels rise before meals and tell the body that it is time to eat. Ghrelin levels increase during pregnancy and are elevated in individuals with Prader-Willi Syndrome, which is character-ized by hyperphagia. Several other gastrointestinal hormones are anorectic and decrease appetite. These hormones include peptide tyrosine tyrosine (PYY), pancreatic polypeptide, oxyntomodu-lin, amylin, glucagon, glucagon-like peptide-1, and glucagon-like peptide-2.[1] PYY, for example, is a satiety signal that acts in the brain. PYY levels increase approximately 15 minutes after eating. PYY is secreted in the small intestine, and the concentration increases distally along the bowel. Individuals who eat very quickly may consume large quantities before the body has time to send satiety signals to the brain and may benefit from techniques to promote slower eating habits.

Hormonal regulation and energy homeostasis are sensitive to factors like sleep and stress, which may also contribute to obesity. Over the past few decades, sleep duration has decreased in children and adults and has coincided with the rise in obesity. Inadequate sleep causes several metabolic changes that can promote weight gain, including decreased glucose tolerance, decreased insulin sensitivity, elevated sympathovagal balance, increased evening cortisol levels, increased ghrelin levels, and decreased leptin levels.[2] These alterations ultimately increase appetite and decrease energy expenditure, which, when combined with more time to eat, are obesogenic. Individuals who are overweight or obese are also at risk for obstructive sleep apnea, which disrupts sleep and is associated with insulin resistance, which also promotes obesity. Poor sleep also appears to be related to increased intake of certain types of foods, particularly carbohydrates and more unhealthy foods. These cravings are associated with higher ghrelin levels. Counseling families on sleep hygiene to ensure adequate, quality sleep can help decrease the hormonal derangements that arise from insufficient sleep.

Stress also causes higher levels of cortisol, which increases food intake. The hypothalamus-pituitary-adrenal axis plays a key role in the stress response. During times of stress, the hypothala-mus releases corticotropin-releasing hormone, which stimulates the anterior pituitary to release adrenocorticotropic hormone (ACTH). ACTH stimulates the adrenal gland to release cortisol. The effect of cortisol is easily seen in patients who start immunosuppression with steroids for underlying medical conditions. These patients demonstrate a significant increase in appetite and often gain weight rapidly. Similarly, individuals with a high cortisol response to stress increase food intake, particularly of highly palatable foods.[3] Stress eating is a recognized phenomenon and appears to act through reward pathways in the brain. High cortisol levels also increase visceral fat stores and are associated with other metabolic abnormalities, such as resistance to insulin and leptin. Helping patients learn to cope with stress is important for stress-induced or emotional eaters.

Several other neuroendocrine hormones are involved in energy regulation. Leptin is an impor-tant messenger of energy status and communicates the energy setpoint to the hypothalamus. Leptin levels correlate with body adiposity and decrease while fasting, leading to the starvation response, with effects such as decreased resting energy expenditure and increased vagal tone and gastric motility.[4] In other words, low leptin levels stimulate eating, whereas high leptin levels sig-nal satiety or sufficient energy reserve. Problems with leptin signaling lead to increased appetite and energy storage. Individuals who are leptin deficient exhibit food foraging behavior and benefit from leptin replacement therapy. Simple obesity is associated with a state of relative leptin resis-tance that may be related to high levels of insulin. Notably during puberty and pregnancy, leptin and insulin levels are both elevated and intertwined because these are times of insulin resistance and higher insulin levels, leading to increased fat stores. Leptin levels rise as expected with the increase in adiposity, but there also appears to be leptin resistance that then promotes building energy stores. Once the body has reached adulthood or is postpartum, leptin levels fall and insu-lin levels decrease. Although this interplay between insulin and leptin may be beneficial during puberty and pregnancy, it becomes maladaptive for the overweight or obese individual and causes even more weight gain.

Leptin is secreted by fat cells and acts on the leptin receptor in the arcuate nucleus of the hypothalamus. The arcuate nucleus promotes orexigenic or eating behavior through agouti-related protein and neuropeptide Y but promotes anorexigenic or appetite suppression through pro-opiomelanocortin and cocaine- and amphetamine-related transcript. Pro-opiomelanocortin is a precursor for several peptides that affect weight, including ACTH and α-melanocyte-stimulating hormone, which acts on the melanocortin 4 receptor. Mutations in melanocortin 4 receptor or other parts of these pathways may be seen in early-onset morbid obesity. Other neurotransmitters are also involved in weight regulation, including gamma-aminobutyric acid, dopamine, serotonin, and histamine. Several medications that act in the brain, such as psychiatric and antiepileptic medications, appear to affect levels of these neurotransmitters, increasing appetite and promoting weight gain.

The endocannabinoid system also plays a role in energy regulation. Two cannabinoid receptors have been discovered, which are known as CB1 and CB2. Several endocannabinoids are ligands for these receptors with anandamide and 2-arachidonoylglycerol being the best understood. The endocannabinoid system works centrally and peripherally through interactions with the hypothalamus, the reward system in corticolimbic areas, leptin, ghrelin, satiety hormones, and other parts of the body including the pancreas, adipose tissue, and skeletal muscle. Studies show that CB1 blockade leads to decreased food intake and body weight while improving lipid metabolism and insulin sensitivity.[5] Rimonabant is a CB1r antagonist that had been approved in Europe as an anti-obesity medication but was withdrawn from the market secondary to psychiatric side effects. Research is being conducted with newer CB1 antagonists that act selectively on the periphery, which may limit psychiatric adverse events.

Finally, the thyroid axis is a pathway often blamed as a cause of obesity because of its function in energy homeostasis. The hypothalamus secretes thyrotropin-releasing hormone, which stimulates the pituitary gland to secrete thyroid-stimulating hormone. Thyroid-stimulating hormone stimulates the thyroid to produce thyroxine and triiodothyronine, which affect body metabolism. Individuals with hypothyroidism will have a lower metabolic rate and benefit from replacement therapy. However, treatment for hypothyroidism may be associated with weight loss of only 5 to 10 pounds. Although hypothyroidism is easy to treat with a pill, it is not as common or as significant a contributor to obesity as an obese patient might hope.

Although many body systems are involved in weight regulation to some degree, the brain, the gastrointestinal system, and the endocrine system are the key players in energy homeostasis. Weight gain due to some problems may be readily treatable, such as in the case of hypothyroidism. However, treating obesity resulting from distortions in the brain-gut-endocrine signaling pathway or from stress eating is much more challenging. Understanding the complexity of the relationships of the different body systems, their signaling pathways, and possible contributing abnormalities can help us to better tailor successful interventions for our patients.

References

1. Karra E, Batterham RL. The role of gut hormones in the regulation of body weight and energy homeostasis. *Mol Cell Endocrinol*. 2010;316:120-128.
2. Van Cauter E, Knutson K. Sleep and the epidemic of obesity in children and adults. *Eur J Endocrinol*. 2008;159(Suppl 1):S59-S66.
3. Adam T, Epel E. Stress, eating and the reward system. *Physiol Behav*. 2007;91:449-458.
4. Bereket A, Kiess W, Lustig RH, et al. Hypothalamic obesity in children. *Obes Rev*. 2012;13:780-798.
5. Bermudez-Silva F, Cardinal P, Cota D. The role of the endocannabinoid system in the neuroendocrine regulation of energy balance. *J Psychopharmacol*. 2012;26:114-124.

QUESTION

OBESITY SEEMS TO RUN IN FAMILIES. WHAT GENETIC FACTORS CONTRIBUTE TO THE DEVELOPMENT OF OBESITY? WHEN SHOULD I SEND AN OVERWEIGHT CHILD FOR EVALUATION FOR A GENETIC SYNDROME?

Patrika Tsai, MD

Genetics is one of the many factors that contribute to obesity. Twin, family, and adoption studies suggest 40% to 70% heritability of body mass index (BMI).[1] Several genome-wide association studies have identified multiple genetic polymorphisms that predispose people to weight gain in cases of common obesity. The strongest of these is the fat mass and obesity-associated risk allele, which is associated with weight gain of 3 to 4 kg.[2] Individuals may have more than one of these single nucleotide polymorphisms, which are single base changes in the DNA that may increase susceptibility to obesity. Copy number variants (CNVs), which are also called *genomic structural variants*, are another genetic phenomenon that can affect BMI. CNVs are deletions or duplications of chromosomal material. Deletion of a segment at the 16p11.2 locus, for example, is associated with severe, early-onset obesity and developmental delay.

Epigenetics is also being shown to play a role in BMI regulation. Epigenetics examines heritable changes in gene expression caused by mechanisms such as DNA methylation, histone modification, or chromatin-modifying proteins effects rather than alterations in the DNA sequence itself. Many of these changes occur in utero and in the neonatal period. One example of DNA methylation involvement is Prader-Willi syndrome. Prader-Willi syndrome is characterized by hyperphagia, developmental delay, intellectual disability, hypotonia, and hypogonadism. Children with Prader-Willi often have problems with failure to thrive initially, but they later exhibit polyphagia. Individuals with Prader-Willi do not receive a paternal copy of the region 15q11-q13. This region is inactivated by methylation on the maternal copy.

Another example of epigenetics is the "natural experiment" of the Dutch famine during World War II. During this time, food rations were limited to 400 to 800 calories per day. Researchers have studied the cohort of individuals born under these severe conditions to understand the in utero effects of maternal undernutrition. These individuals have higher rates of cardiovascular

Huang JS, ed. *Curbside Consultation in
Pediatric Obesity: 49 Clinical Questions* (pp 17-19).
© 2014 Taylor & Francis Group

Table 5-1
Characteristic Findings in
Genetic Syndromes Associated With Obesity

Albright's hereditary osteodystrophy	Short stature, short fourth and fifth metacarpals, intellectual disability, developmental delay
Alström syndrome	Cone-rod retinal dystrophy, hearing loss
Bardet-Biedl syndrome	Retinitis pigmentosa, kidney dysfunction, polydactyly, short stature, developmental delay
Börjeson-Forssman-Lehmann syndrome	Gynecomastia, hypogonadism, intellectual disability
Fragile X syndrome	Macroorchidism, intellectual disability, developmental delay
Maternal uniparental disomy chromosome 14	Hypotonia, intellectual disability, developmental delay
Prader-Willi syndrome	Short stature, hypotonia, hypogonadism, intellectual disability, developmental delay
Rapid-onset obesity with hypothalamic dysregulation, hypoventilation, and autonomic dysregulation (ROHHAD) syndrome	Autonomic dysregulation, neuroendocrine tumors

disease, type 2 diabetes, obesity, and breast cancer. Interestingly, the children of these individuals also have higher rates of obesity, showing transgenerational effects of maternal nutrition.[3]

In some cases, obesity can be traced to mutations in a single gene, which is termed *monogenic obesity*. Monogenic obesity with typical morbid obesity by age 2 years is rare. Monogenic obesity may be nonsyndromic or syndromic and is characterized by severe, early-onset obesity by age 5 years with a BMI greater than the 99th percentile or greater than 3 standard deviations. Nonsyndromic forms of monogenic obesity include mutations in leptin and leptin receptors. Leptin is secreted by adipocytes and plays a key role in energy homeostasis. Individuals with leptin deficiency benefit from leptin replacement therapy. Mutations in genes in the melanocortin pathway, including pro-opiomelanocortin, also cause nonsyndromic obesity. Pro-opiomelanocortin is a precursor for several proteins involved in weight regulation, including adrenocorticotropic hormone and α-melanocyte-stimulating hormone, which acts on the melanocortin 4 receptor. Melanocortin 4 receptor mutations are the most common currently known cause of monogenic obesity. The existence of monogenic obesity demonstrates the lack of redundancy in some pathways involved in weight regulation. Syndromes associated with obesity include Prader-Willi syndrome and maternal uniparental disomy chromosome 14 (Table 5-1). Ciliopathies or syndromes associated with ciliary dysfunction also are associated with obesity and include Bardet-Biedl and Alström syndromes and Albright's hereditary osteodystrophy. Some syndromes have distinctive characteristics. Children may show classic findings such as hypotonia and poor feeding followed by early-onset obesity in Prader-Willi syndrome. Children with Albright's hereditary osteodystrophy have short fourth and fifth metacarpals. Such findings can help in establishing the diagnosis of certain genetic syndromes associated with morbid obesity.

Although pharmacologic treatment for obesity associated with genetic causes is available in a limited number of cases, such as leptin deficiency, knowing there is a genetic cause for their child's obesity may be helpful for parents who often become frustrated or feel blamed for their child's weight and may also be important for the treatment of other associated abnormalities such as endocrinopathies. Monogenic obesity is often characterized by food-foraging behavior. Such a description from a parent along with early-onset obesity warrants referral to genetics or an obesity clinic for further workup. Evaluation and testing for a genetic syndrome should be considered in children with severe early-onset obesity with or without findings concerning for obesity-associated syndromes. Such findings may include hypotonia, hypogonadism, short stature, polydactyly, developmental delay, and intellectual or learning disability. If a child shows a rapid increase in weight, you should also consider pituitary disorders that may be treatable. The differential diagnoses include brain tumors such as craniopharyngioma, endocrine disorders such as hypothyroidism, growth hormone deficiency, and Cushing's disease. Testing with array comparative genomic hybridization analysis can detect CNVs and some deletions causing Prader-Willi syndrome.[2] Other targeted genetic testing can be performed for syndromic obesity with classic findings such as Albright's hereditary osteodystrophy.

Our knowledge about the genetic and epigenetic causes of obesity is increasing rapidly with the availability of techniques like array comparative genomic hybridization analysis. Although some risk alleles may contribute to only a few kilograms of weight gain, monogenic obesity is associated with morbid obesity. Genetics and epigenetics may therefore have varying degrees of significance in a given individual's risk for obesity.

References

1. Maes HH, Neale MC, Eaves LJ. Genetic and environmental factors in relative body weight and human adiposity. *Behav Genet.* 1997;27:325-351.
2. Phan-Hug F, Beckmann JS, Jacquemont S. Genetic testing in patients with obesity. *Best Pract Res Clin Endocrinol Metab.* 2012;26:133-143.
3. Veenendaal MVE, Painter RC, de Rooij SR, et al. Transgenerational effects of prenatal exposure to the 1944–45 Dutch famine. *BJOG.* 2013;120(5):548-553.

QUESTION

WHAT MAJOR SOCIAL FACTORS CONTRIBUTE TO CHILDHOOD OBESITY, AND HOW CAN CLINICIANS AND CAREGIVERS ALTER THEIR IMPACT?

Abby L. Braden, PhD and Kyung E. Rhee, MD, MSc, MA

Rates of childhood obesity in the United States dramatically increased during the 1980s and 1990s, resulting in what has been called an epidemic of childhood obesity. Unfortunately, ethnic minority children have been disproportionately affected by the obesity crisis. According to the 1999-2010 National Health and Nutrition Examination Survey, 21.2% of Hispanic youth and 24.3% of non-Hispanic Black youth are obese (body mass index [BMI] greater than the 95th percentile) compared with only 14% of non-Hispanic White youth.[1] These rates mirror America's poverty rates, with 27.4% of African Americans and 26.6% of Hispanics living in poverty compared with 9.9% of non-Hispanic Whites.[2] Exposure to poverty in early childhood predicts a higher BMI trajectory from ages 9 to 17 years.[3] Parent level of education, parent occupation, and family income are socioeconomic indicators that are inversely associated with child risk for obesity.[4] High levels of family stress, type of social connections, and problematic parent feeding practices are some underlying mechanisms that help explain the relationship between socioeconomic status (SES) and obesity in children. Clinicians working with overweight children need to be aware of these social factors so they can address these issues with their families and provide the most effective treatments.

Multiple factors are likely contributing to why children from lower SES are at a higher risk for obesity. First, these families often experience chronic social adversities, including food and housing insecurity, lack of access to health care, poorer school systems, and exposure to unsafe neighborhoods and environmental contaminants. Children in these environments are also likely to be exposed to abuse or neglect, intimate partner violence, parental incarceration, maternal depression, and parent substance abuse. Unfortunately, caregivers in these situations are often overwhelmed with pressing financial, psychological, and interpersonal concerns that interfere with their ability to focus on making sure their children are eating right and being physically active. Economic

Huang JS, ed. *Curbside Consultation in Pediatric Obesity: 49 Clinical Questions* (pp 21-24).
© 2014 Taylor & Francis Group

concerns and the stress of everyday living in the midst of poorer neighborhoods with greater numbers of fast food restaurants, fewer grocery stores, and limited recreational facilities can all interact and make it difficult for caregivers to have the time and wherewithal to cook a healthy meal or spend time doing something physically active. In addition to the external pressures of living in poverty, stress can act internally to affect one's hypothalamic-pituitary-adrenal axis and release excess amounts of cortisol. Foods high in fat and sugar help reduce the hypothalamic-pituitary-adrenal response to repeated stressors and decrease the amount of cortisol released.[5,6] As a result, over time, people learn that these foods help them feel better (becoming comfort foods) when they are under high levels of stress. Chronic stressors, in conjunction with biological responses, may explain the high prevalence of obesity among youth who are in lower SES groups.

A child's immediate social network may also help explain the relationship between low SES and obesity. Social interactions can play a powerful role in the development of children's eating habits, physical activity levels, and overall body weight. In 2007, Christakis and Fowler[7] published a groundbreaking study describing the "spread of obesity" through social connections. They found that a person's chance of becoming obese increased by 57% if that person had a friend who became obese during the study period. The authors suggested that perceptions of health behavior norms, in addition to shared eating environments, physical activity habits, and leisure time behaviors, may all lead to the "spread of obesity" between friends and family. For example, if a child's family members or friends preferred processed fast food and ate few fruits and vegetables, a child would be highly likely to imitate these behaviors and assume these unhealthy eating practices, thereby increasing his or her risk for obesity. Although children were not included in this study, these results are relevant and demonstrate that, aside from biological influences, one's social network could have a significant impact on obesity rates. These findings also suggest that additional attention should be paid to one's social network and the eating and activity behaviors they engage in.

Specific parent feeding practices among lower SES groups may also contribute to elevated rates of obesity in children. Breastfeeding is thought to protect against the development of obesity, possibly through the content of the breast milk or the promotion of self-regulatory abilities in the children. However, breastfeeding is less common among women with lower SES, and particularly among some ethnic minority groups. Furthermore, in several ethnic groups, mothers tend to believe that a heavy baby is an indicator of a healthy baby, an expectation that may encourage overfeeding and eventual overeating by children. Other parent feeding practices can also promote child obesity by inadvertently teaching children to eat for reasons other than hunger. For example, some parents reward their children with food (eg, offering a cookie if the child behaves in the grocery store), and some parents suggest food as a means of coping with negative emotions. Consequently, children may learn to eat food when their body is not truly hungry, thereby contributing to overeating and obesity.

Given what we know about the social factors influencing child eating and activity behaviors, an important first step is to increase awareness of these factors with parents, highlighting obesity as a problem of our society and not as a sign of weakness or failure. Clinicians can validate how difficult it can be for parents to help their children improve health behaviors in the midst of any life stressors they are experiencing. This initial step can be useful toward reducing parental or child self-blame and may encourage active participation in subsequent discussions about how to make eating and activity changes to combat these social factors.

As you begin to have these discussions with your patients and families, you can implement a variety of strategies to help them become more aware of these social influences at work around them.

1. *Address the impact of stress and discuss unhealthy social environments.* Clinicians can acknowledge the high level of stress endured by families of a low SES background, identifying this as a barrier to healthy nutrition and exercise. Clinicians can simultaneously explain the importance of the overall family and social environment on the child, with the intention of motivating

1	2	3	4	5
Starving	Hungry	Just Right	Full	Stuffed
You skipped a meal. You have a headache, can't focus, and feel grumpy.	It has been several hours since you last ate. You are getting ready for your next meal.	You are not hungry anymore, but you are not overly full either.	You ate too much. Your stomach is big and you feel full. Exercising would not be comfortable right now.	You ate far too much. Your stomach is big and feels sick.

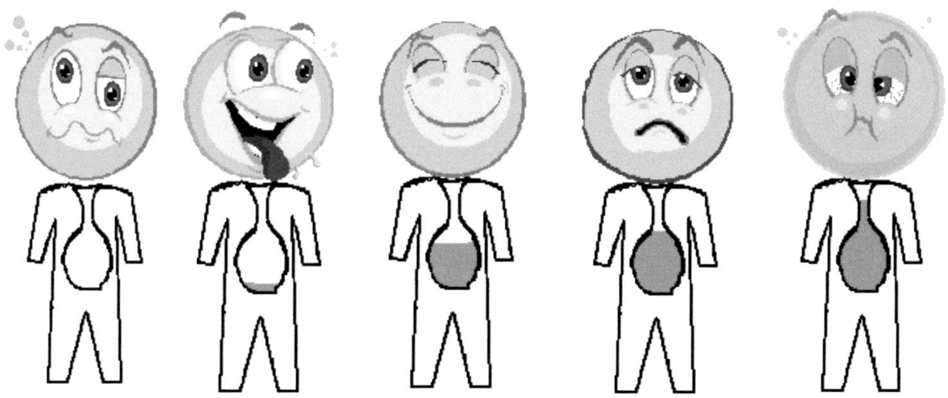

Figure 6-1. Hunger meter.

parents to engage in and model more healthy behaviors. It may be helpful to ask how the family responds to stress, brainstorm adaptive coping strategies, and make referrals for psychological assessment or treatment when necessary. Explaining how eating high-fat comfort food is a natural response to stress may help families identify this behavior when it occurs and try to bypass it with other stress-reducing behaviors, such as taking a walk.

2. *Provide education on healthy feeding practices.* Teaching parents basic knowledge and tips about weight, eating, and physical activity may be a key component in treating these families. Clinicians can talk about the consequences of specific unhelpful feeding strategies (like using food as a reward), and encourage parents to help their children to eat in response to genuine feelings of hunger. Providers may introduce the concept of a "hunger meter" as a way to teach children to monitor their feelings of hunger and satiety. Using a visual representation of a hunger meter, parents can be encouraged to talk to their children about physical signs of hunger and fullness (Figure 6-1). Finally, addressing barriers around breastfeeding and myths that a healthy baby is a heavy baby may help families adopt healthier feeding styles.

3. *Become an advocate for child obesity prevention and treatment.* Prevention efforts may be a critical component in the fight against childhood obesity, a strategy that may preferentially target and benefit minority groups who are at highest risk. Clinicians can advocate for social policies that increase access or decrease exposure to unhealthy foods and environments by contacting local and regional politicians. They can also aim to promote changes on a larger level by connecting with their local chapter of the American Academy of Pediatrics. Advocacy may be one of the most effective methods of reducing the impact of social factors on childhood obesity (see Question 49).

References

1. United States Census Bureau. Poverty. http://www.census.gov/hhes/www/poverty/. Revised January 13, 2014. Accessed March 14, 2013.
2. Ogden CL, Carroll MD, Kit BK, Flegal KM. Prevalence of obesity and trends in body mass index among US children and adolescents, 1999-2010. *JAMA*. 2012;307(5):483-490.
3. Wells NM, Evans GW, Beavis A, Ong AD. Early childhood poverty, cumulative risk exposure, and body mass index trajectories through young adulthood. *Am J Public Health*. 2010;100(12):2507-2512.
4. Shrewsbury V, Wardle J. Socioeconomic status and adiposity in childhood: a systematic review of cross-sectional studies 1990-2005. *Obesity (Silver Spring)*. 2008;16(2):275-284.
5. Dallman M, Pecoraro N, la Fleur SE. Chronic stress and comfort foods: self-medication and abdominal obesity. *Brain Behav Immun*. 2005;19(4):275-280.
6. Rutledge T, Linden W. To eat or not to eat: affective and physiological mechanisms in the stress-eating relationship. *J Behav Med*. 1998;21(3):221-240.
7. Christakis NA, Fowler JH. The spread of obesity in a large social network over 32 years. *N Engl J Med*. 2007;357:370-379.

QUESTION

HOW DOES THE MOTHER'S NUTRITIONAL STATUS DURING PREGNANCY CONTRIBUTE TO OR PREVENT THE DEVELOPMENT OF OBESITY?

Andrea J. Sharma, PhD and Stefanie N. Hinkle, PhD

Disclaimer: The findings and conclusions in this report are those of the authors and not necessarily those of the Centers for Disease Control and Prevention.

The rise in obesity has primarily been attributed to overconsumption of energy-rich diets and lifestyles with reduced energy expenditures. However, it is now recognized that events in utero have long-term influences on disease risk later in life through a phenomenon known as *early life programming.*[1] Fetal growth is complex and depends on both genetics and the intrauterine environment. In response to the intrauterine environment, the developing fetus makes adaptations to maximize immediate chance for survival. These adaptations, which can include permanent changes in structure, physiology, and hormonal axes, can increase risk for disease as one gets older. Maternal nutritional status prior to and during pregnancy is an important determinant of the intrauterine environment affecting nutrient supply for fetal growth and development. Overnutrition, as a result of maternal obesity or excess gestational weight gain, and undernutrition, from inadequate maternal diet or impaired transport of the nutrients to the fetus, have been linked to an increased risk for obesity in the child. Here we summarize evidence for these associations and discuss the complexities given the shared postnatal lifestyle between mothers and their children. Because obesity in childhood tends to track into adulthood, maternal transmission of obesity may lead to an intergenerational cycle of maternal and child obesity. We highlight opportunities to break this cycle.

Approximately 1 in 3 women of reproductive age in the United States are obese (body mass index [BMI] ≥30 kg/m²). Obesity causes low-grade systemic inflammation, increased oxidative stress, increased insulin resistance, hyperglycemia, hyperinsulinemia, and hypertriglyceridemia.[1,2] During pregnancy, the metabolic dysregulation caused by obesity is exacerbated as a result of the concomitant increase in insulin resistance and hyperlipidemia that occurs to mobilize nutrients

Huang JS, ed. *Curbside Consultation in Pediatric Obesity: 49 Clinical Questions* (pp 25-28).
© 2014 Taylor & Francis Group

to the growing fetus. For some, these metabolic changes result in gestational diabetes mellitus (GDM). Whereas only approximately 5% of pregnancies are affected by GDM annually, obese or severely obese women are 4 to 8 times more likely to develop GDM compared with normal-weight women. Many observational studies show that children born to obese mothers are more likely to be obese than those born to normal-weight mothers, even in the absence of maternal GDM.[1,2]

The metabolic dysregulation of maternal obesity during pregnancy may contribute to the development of child obesity in several ways. Fetal growth is directly affected by the intrauterine environment of obese mothers by exposing the developing fetus to excessive nutrient supply in the forms of glucose, amino acids, and triglycerides.[1-3] The fetal pancreas and liver are stimulated to secrete more insulin and insulin-like growth factors, both growth-promoting hormones leading to excess fetal growth and increased storage of lipids in adipose tissue. The increase in adipose tissue may be a compensatory adaptation, so excess lipids are not stored in metabolic organs, leading to their dysfunction.[3] Consequently, obese mothers are more likely to have infants born large (birth weight > 4000 g) with greater fat mass than those of nonobese mothers. These larger infants tend to continue on this growth trajectory, being twice as likely to be obese by preschool age.[1,2] While GDM may carry additional risk for child obesity, much of the association is explained by maternal obesity, a more prevalent condition.[1]

The intrauterine environment associated with maternal obesity may also increase child obesity risk through developmental programming of metabolic systems.[1-3] For example, development of hypothalamic and associated neuroendocrine tissues is regulated, in part, by insulin and leptin, which are higher among obese mothers and their infants.[2] The hypothalamus plays a key role in regulating appetite and eating behaviors by responding to signals including leptin and insulin. In animal studies, fetal hyperinsulinemia and hyperleptinemia can induce morphological changes in hypothalamic structure and affect later sensitivity to insulin and leptin signaling resulting in hyperphagia and altered food choices.[2,3] Similarly, fetal hyperinsulinemia has been shown to alter insulin receptor profiles in developing skeletal muscle, adipocytes, pancreas, and liver tissues. Modification in epigenetic regulation of gene expression has also been observed in these tissues. If permanent, impairment of leptin- and insulin-signaling pathways may have long-term implications for eating behaviors, energy balance, and glucose-insulin homeostasis.[2,3] In addition, the altered body composition and excess fat mass developed in utero is an early source of inflammation and oxidative stress, increasing risk for long-term insulin resistance, metabolic dysfunction, and obesity.

Although maternal obesity is more strongly associated with child obesity, excess weight gain during pregnancy is also a source of excess nutrient supply contributing to increased fetal growth and perhaps developmental programming through pathways similar to obesity. Guidelines for appropriate gestational weight gain depend on the mother's pregravid BMI; lean mothers are recommended to gain more weight and obese mothers less. Despite recommendations, only 30% to 40% of mothers gain appropriately.[1] Mothers exceeding recommendations are more likely to have children with higher birth weights and greater adiposity.[1,2] Even with excess weight gain, the proportional change in weight is significantly less for an obese mother compared with a leaner mother. Thus, the influence of excess gestational weight gain is stronger among mothers who were not obese prior to conception.[1] Likewise excess gestational weight gain early in pregnancy may be more strongly associated with later child obesity because of the timing of the development of fetal organ systems. However, more research is needed because few studies measure serial weight gain patterns throughout pregnancy.

In contrast to maternal obesity, approximately 3% of women of reproductive age in the United States are underweight (BMI < 18.5 kg/m²). Studies of women pregnant during a famine suggest that acute undernutrition early in pregnancy also increases the risk of obesity in children. However, intervention trials in which food (protein and energy) supplementation was provided to chronically undernourished mothers during pregnancy observed no differences in later obesity among the children. Similarly, interventional trials in which micronutrients such as iron, folic acid, zinc, or vitamin A were provided during pregnancy reported mixed findings about subsequent adiposity among the children. These trials have limited generalizability because they took place in developing countries with a low prevalence of obesity; thus, further research is needed.[2] Currently, evidence that inadequate gestational weight gain increases risk of child obesity regardless of pregravid BMI is limited.

Although not a direct indicator of maternal nutritional status, maternal smoking during pregnancy increases the risk of child obesity.[2,4] Maternal smoking impairs nutrient transport and is a known risk factor for intrauterine growth retardation. The vasoconstrictive properties of nicotine reduce oxygenation of the placenta and blood supply to the fetus. Similar to obesity, smoking increases markers of inflammation and oxidative stress. Nicotine also suppresses appetite, which may reduce nutrient intake by the mother. In adults, nicotine withdrawal results in hyperphagia and weight gain. Interestingly, studies suggest that infants exposed to smoking in utero have accelerated postnatal weight gain.[4]

It is difficult to separate intrauterine from postnatal influences on child obesity because of shared genetics, family lifestyles, and the presence of other risk factors associated with both maternal and child obesity. For example, children's dietary and physical activity patterns tend to resemble those of their mothers, as do the adverse influences of social status. Obese mothers as well as mothers who smoke are less likely to initiate breastfeeding or they breastfeed for a shorter time compared with normal-weight or nonsmoking mothers.[2] Breastfeeding is hypothesized to have a protective effect on child obesity through learned satiety or bioactive factors in breast milk that might modulate growth. Sibling studies, however, support an association between maternal nutritional status and child obesity independent of these potential confounding factors.[1,2]

Many opportunities exist to break the cycle of maternal and child obesity. Obesity and smoking are known risk factors for adverse pregnancy outcomes. Before women become pregnant, health care providers can provide evidence-based risk screening, health promotion, and interventions to help them achieve a healthy, normal weight and to quit smoking. Dietary and physical activity interventions during pregnancy can control diabetes and may prevent excess gestational weight gain or postpartum weight retention, which can affect the next pregnancy. For infants and children, guidance includes supporting mothers to exclusively breastfeed to about 6 months of age with appropriate complementary feeding and breastfeeding thereafter, providing nutrition education for an age-appropriate balanced diet, encouraging daily physical activity, and conducting regular growth monitoring. Adolescence may be an overlooked window of opportunity to break the cycle of maternal and child obesity. As the next generation of mothers, adolescent girls may need targeted interventions to reduce obesity and improve lifestyle behaviors; making these changes prior to their reproductive years may confer lasting effects on obesity prevention for future generations. Furthermore, obesity and teen pregnancy share many common socioecological determinants, such as inadequate access to health services and socioeconomic disadvantage. Because teen pregnancy increases these risk of adverse pregnancy outcomes and may contribute to a lifetime of obesity through excess gestational weight gain and postpartum weight retention, additional benefits may come from providing contraceptive counseling to adolescent girls. Thus, to improve the health of our next generation of mothers and break the vicious cycle of obesity, continued outreach is needed to educate and encourage adolescent girls to maintain a healthy diet, meet physical activity guidelines, and quit or never start smoking well before they even consider having a family.

Maternal and child obesity are common public health challenges. Intergenerational programming effects further increase the scale of these challenges. Public health initiatives aimed at preventing obesity and improving the nutritional status and lifestyle of women of reproductive age, and even before they reach reproductive capability, are important for the health of future generations.

Acknowledgment

This research was supported in part by the Intramural Research Program of the NIH, Eunice Kennedy Shriver National Institute of Child Health and Human Development.

References

1. O'Reilly JR, Reynolds RM. The risk of maternal obesity to the long-term health of the offspring. *Clin Endocrinol (Oxf)*. 2013;78(1):9-16.
2. Fall CH. Evidence for the intra-uterine programming of adiposity in later life. *Ann Hum Biol*. 2011;38(4):410-428.
3. Alfaradhi MZ, Ozanne SE. Developmental programming in response to maternal overnutrition. *Front Genet*. 2011;2:27.
4. Oken E, Levitan EB, Gillman MW. Maternal smoking during pregnancy and child overweight: systematic review and meta-analysis. *Int J Obes (Lond)*. 2008;32(2):201-210.

QUESTION

8

IS THERE ANY RELATIONSHIP BETWEEN SLEEP AND THE DEVELOPMENT AND PREVENTION OF OBESITY?

David Gozal, MD

There is only one thing people like that is good for them; a good night's sleep. —E.W. Howe

In recent years, evidence has accumulated on the potentially important role of sleep and sleep disorders in either promoting the onset of or aggravating existing obesity and its complications. Conversely, the role of obesity in the pathophysiology of sleep disorders, particularly sleep-disordered breathing, has also been evidenced. The evidence on the bilateral and mutual interactions linking sleep and obesity in children is briefly reviewed herein.

Societies in general, and more particularly technologically driven societies, have transformed and generated an increasingly demanding lifestyle. Such changes in lifestyle have in turn markedly altered sleep patterns and duration, even in children, and could also reflect trends in parenting approaches. For example, the concept of afternoon naps is virtually absent today, even among younger children. The progressive decrements in sleep duration and in sleep regularity over a period spanning several decades have been accompanied by the aforementioned surge in the prevalence of childhood obesity. An increasingly growing body of evidence suggests the existence of a strong association between sleep duration and obesity. However, associations between body mass index (BMI) and bedtime, bedtime irregularity, or even technology in the bedroom have also been proposed as underlying the increases in obesity rates. Furthermore, the link between sleep and obesity could be mediated by socioeconomic status.

The potential biological correlates of such associations have been partially uncovered. Overall, research to date supports the concept that inadequate amounts of sleep, as well as circadian alterations in food consumption and rhythmicity, lead to alterations in some of the neuropeptides that regulate appetite. In particular, increased levels of ghrelin, reduced levels of leptin, reduced central biological activity of orexin, and other complex alterations in hypothalamic pathways have been demonstrated in association with altered sleep, thereby promoting increased food intake.

Huang JS, ed. *Curbside Consultation in Pediatric Obesity: 49 Clinical Questions* (pp 29-31).
© 2014 Taylor & Francis Group

Although the overall data are supportive of an association between short sleep duration and an increased risk for obesity, studies are somewhat conflicting, albeit not irreconcilably so, for any of the age groups examined. For example, multiple studies have identified a significant contribution of sleep duration to obesity risk in adults, but such findings have not always been reproduced. Lack of universal reproducibility may reflect either methodological issues in defining short sleep as compared with insufficient sleep or multiple confounders in the propensity for obesity that can start early in life. In a cross-sectional and longitudinal study, only subjects with short sleep duration exhibited highly disinhibited eating behavior and low dietary calcium intake and were at risk for developing significantly higher BMI compared with the reference cohort among both sexes. During the 6-year follow-up period, the high-risk adult subjects were significantly more likely to gain weight and develop obesity criteria. To further clarify these issues, intervention trials aiming to establish whether prolongation of sleep will improve metabolic and ponderal indices have been initiated in adults.

Although studies support that the strength of the association between sleep duration and obesity is stronger in children and adolescents and declines over time, the strength of the association can be somewhat challenged, even in children. Furthermore, some degree of predisposition for the existence of such association has been advanced because sleep-associated changes in BMI appear to be primarily affecting children whose BMIs are already elevated or children with specific genetic backgrounds. Another important issue worthy of mention is the fact that the vast majority of sleep studies in children to date have relied on subjective estimates of sleep duration. Furthermore, the impact of the variability of sleep schedules on BMI has not been extensively explored, and the effects of specific sleep patterns on metabolic homeostasis in children are unknown, even if irregular sleep schedules as a group appear to impose a higher metabolic burden. Studies assessing sleep duration and obesity relationships are further hampered by the obstacles and inherent challenges of measuring sleep duration in a natural environment; therefore, most studies thus far have relied on parental reports of sleep duration. However, parental reports generally overestimate sleep duration in their children. In studies using actigraphy to record sleep, the vast majority have relied on limited-duration recordings that preclude accurate assessments of regularity of sleep patterns and stability of any specific phenotype. Furthermore, longitudinal sleep studies are scarce, and the disparity in subject characteristics across such studies further adds to the limitations of our current understanding. In addition, delineation of normal sleep duration in children is still elusive. For example, some authors approached the potential confounders in existing studies (eg, sex distribution, sample size, sampling frequency and duration) and yet applied arbitrary cutoff values for defining short sleep in children. In contrast, other authors employed an arbitrary cutoff value (ie, ≤ 10 hours per night).

As with adults, the heterogeneity of the published associations between sleep duration and obesity reported in children range from absence of any association to a negative linear trend or to a U-shaped relationship, and such discrepancies may simply reflect sampling bias or overcontrolling for certain variables. We should remember that sleep duration and body weight are both determined by a multitude of factors, such as genetic, sociodemographic, socioeconomic, familial (eg, family structure, overweight parent), and individual (eg, health behavior, health status) factors, and thus studies evaluating associations between sleep and weight status should incorporate potential biases, confounders, and covariates in the interpretation of any findings. Regardless of the aforementioned limitations, studies evaluating the association of sleep with BMI generally demonstrate a 1.5- to 2-fold increase (odds ratio, 1.15 to 11) of being a shorter sleeper if obesity is present.

Interventions aiming to modify sleep patterns in children may be difficult to implement, particularly considering that both sleep regularity and sleep duration are stable traits over long periods of time during childhood. In light of this, the effects of sleep patterns on BMI z-score and on cardiometabolic markers may be difficult to modify if putative interventions are not implemented early in life. Nevertheless, 1 of every 3 obese preschool children and approximately every other obese school-aged child will become obese adults. Thus, notwithstanding our inadequate level of understanding on the relationship between sleep and obesity, every incentive exists to identify those children at higher risk for developing obesity and to consider implementing policies and social initiatives to prolong and regularize sleep.

In this context, the following recommendations should assist in optimizing sleep patterns in children and potentially minimize the impact of this component in the constellation of obesity risk factors:

- Children should maintain regular bedtime and wake-up schedules.

- Children should obtain a minimum of 9.5 to 10 hours of sleep each night.

- Ideally, with the implementation of recommendations 1 and 2, children will wake up on their own at the desired time for school/required events and not require their parents to awaken them each morning.

Suggested Readings

Cappuccio FP, Taggart FM, Kandala NB, et al. Meta-analysis of short sleep duration and obesity in children and adults. *Sleep.* 2008;31(5):619-626.

Chen X, Beydoun MA, Wang Y. Is sleep duration associated with childhood obesity? A systematic review and meta-analysis. *Obesity (Silver Spring).* 2008;16(2):265-274.

Jarrin DC, McGrath JJ, Drake CL. Beyond sleep duration: distinct sleep dimensions are associated with obesity in children and adolescents. *Int J Obes (Lond).* 2013;37(4):552-558.

Matricciani LA, Olds TS, Blunden S, Rigney G, Williams MT. Never enough sleep: a brief history of sleep recommendations for children. *Pediatrics.* 2012;129(3):548-556.

Monasta L, Batty GD, Cattaneo A, et al. Early-life determinants of overweight and obesity: a review of systematic reviews. *Obes Rev.* 2010;11(10):695-708.

Nielsen LS, Danielsen KV, Sørensen TI. Short sleep duration as a possible cause of obesity: critical analysis of the epidemiological evidence. *Obes Rev.* 2010;12(2):78-92.

Spruyt K, Gozal D. The underlying interactome of childhood obesity: the potential role of sleep. *Child Obes.* 2012;8(1):38-42.

Spruyt K, Molfese DL, Gozal D. Sleep duration, sleep regularity, body weight, and metabolic homeostasis in school-aged children. *Pediatrics.* 2011;127(2):e345-e352.

Tauman R, Gozal D. Obesity and obstructive sleep apnea in children. *Paediatr Respir Rev.* 2006;7(4):247-259.

SECTION III

ENVIRONMENT

HOW DOES THE ENVIRONMENT CONTRIBUTE TO THE DEVELOPMENT OF CHILDHOOD OBESITY? HOW DO COMMUNITY INFLUENCES AFFECT CHILDHOOD OBESITY RISK?

Jacqueline Kerr, PhD

For decades, obesity prevention focused on motivating individuals to eat more healthily and to be more active. Such interventions, including physician counseling, often had only short-term effects, and the obesity epidemic is evidence that such an approach remains ineffective. In childhood obesity, parental influences on physical activity and eating were recognized early on, but only in the past decade have larger community influences been considered. Although few intervention studies have tested comprehensive community-based obesity-prevention strategies, Ecological Models of Behavior Change posit that you need to provide individual children with clear goals and behavior-change skills and to encourage family members to adopt healthier habits and support opportunities for health behaviors, that families need to have access to healthy community resources such as fresh fruit markets and recreation centers, that schools should provide healthy food and physical education, and that state and federal agencies should facilitate community change through policies and financial incentives. Despite the lack of evidence in intervention trials, agencies like the Institute of Medicine[1] and the Centers for Disease Control (CDC)[2] have made recommendations that include community-wide approaches to obesity prevention. The latter follows a simple logic (Figure 9-1).

If we reflect on society today compared with 40 years ago, children now may live in communities where it is not perceived as safe to walk to school, where there is no physical education in school, where local parks are places for gangs and drug users, where large roads and cars dominate the landscape, where both parents work and are unable to provide freshly cooked meals at home, where advertisers entice children to eat sugary cereals and beverages with toys and cartoon characters, and where processed foods are cheap and available on every street corner. Although individuals are responsible for the choices they make, the barriers to making healthy choices far outweigh the incentives and cues for more convenient unhealthy behaviors. Physicians can provide advice

Huang JS, ed. *Curbside Consultation in Pediatric Obesity: 49 Clinical Questions* (pp 35-37).
© 2014 Taylor & Francis Group

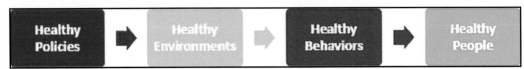

Figure 9-1. CDC's logic model for community strategies to prevent childhood obesity.

to parents and children to be active and eat healthily but must recognize that developing these skills is a complex endeavor and sustaining healthy behavior requires conscious avoidance of many social environments that prompt overeating and inactivity. Physicians can suggest to their patients ways to create supportive home environments, such as fresh fruit on the counter, vegetable snack foods, and active Nintendo Wii games instead of TV, but they must acknowledge that children spend much time outside of the home. Nevertheless, physicians can and should implement obesity screening, serve as role models for their patients, and provide leadership for obesity prevention efforts in their communities by advocating for institutional (eg, child care, school, and worksite), community, and state-level strategies that can improve physical activity and nutrition resources for their patients and their communities (see Question 49).

In 2012, the Institute of Medicine evaluated prior obesity prevention strategies and identified recommendations to accelerate progress. Some strategies are as follows:

- Communities, organizations, community planners, and public health professionals should encourage physical activity by enhancing the physical and built environment (eg, sidewalks and parks), rethinking community design (eg, have houses, schools, and shops in walking distance), and ensuring access to places for activity. Communities and organizations should encourage physical activity by providing and supporting programs designed to increase activity.

- Decision makers in the business community/private sector, in nongovernmental organizations, and at all levels of government should adopt comprehensive strategies to reduce overconsumption of sugar-sweetened beverages. Chain and quick-service restaurants should substantially reduce the number of calories served to children and substantially expand the number of affordable and competitively priced healthier options available for parents to choose from. States and communities should use financial incentives, such as flexible financing or tax credits, streamlined permitting processes, and zoning strategies, to enhance the quality of local food environments, particularly in low-income communities. Incentives should be linked to public health goals in ways that give priority to stores that also commit to health-promoting retail strategies (eg, through placement, promotion, and pricing).

- The food, beverage, restaurant, and media industries should take action to make substantial improvements in their marketing aimed directly at children and adolescents aged 2 to 17 years. All foods and beverages marketed to this age group should support a diet that accords with the *Dietary Guidelines for Americans* to prevent obesity (eg, avoid products high in sugar, fat, and sodium and encourage fruits, vegetables, and whole grains).

- The standards set for foods and beverages marketed to children and adolescents should be widely publicized and easily available to parents and other consumers. They should cover foods and beverages marketed to children and adolescents aged 2 to 17 years and should apply to a broad range of marketing and advertising practices, including digital marketing and the use of licensed characters and toy premiums. Policy makers at the local, state, and federal levels should consider setting mandatory nutritional standards for marketing to this age group.

- Through support from federal and state governments, state and local education agencies and local school districts should ensure that all students in grades kindergarten through 12 have adequate opportunities to engage in 60 minutes of physical activity per school day. This 60-minute goal includes access to and participation in quality physical education.

- All government agencies (federal, state, local, and school district) providing foods and beverages to children and adolescents have a responsibility to provide those in their care with foods and beverages that promote health and learning. The *Dietary Guidelines for Americans* provide specific, science-based recommendations for optimizing dietary intake to prevent disease and promote health.

- Through leadership and guidance from federal and state governments, state and local education agencies should ensure the implementation and monitoring of sequential food literacy and nutrition science education, spanning grades kindergarten through 12, based on the food and nutrition recommendations in the *Dietary Guidelines for Americans*.[3]

The recommendations call for collaborations across many industries and sectors, including health care services. To effect such change, physicians could and should serve on childhood obesity initiatives or coalitions, provide support to school boards developing wellness policies, or provide expertise to local government agencies on public health approaches to obesity prevention. Although this may be difficult to achieve with long clinical hours, practice managers should recognize that physicians will be more effective if they play an active role in their community. The CDC's community strategies guide[2] has links to resources for different strategies and examples of community action.

References

1. Institute of Medicine. *Accelerating Progress in Obesity Prevention: Solving the Weight of the Nation.* May 2012. http://www.iom.edu/~/media/Files/Report%20Files/2012/APOP/APOP_insert.pdf. Accessed November 12, 2013.

2. US Department of Health and Human Services, Centers for Disease Control and Prevention. *Recommended Community Strategies and Measurements to Prevent Obesity in the United States: Implementation and Measurement Guide.* July 2009. http://www.cdc.gov/obesity/downloads/community_strategies_guide.pdf. Accessed November 12, 2013.

3. US Department of Health and Human Services. *Dietary Guidelines for Americans.* http://www.health.gov/dietaryguidelines. Accessed November 12, 2013.

·

I Have Heard About Links Between Obesity and Infectious Agents. How Do Virus Infections Affect the Development of Obesity in Children? How Do Bacteria in the Gut Affect the Development of Obesity in Children?

Richard L. Atkinson, MD

Virus Infections and Obesity

All pediatricians in America are familiar with the sharp upswing in childhood obesity starting in the 1980s. Many in the lay press, politicians, and even obesity experts attribute this increase in obesity to factors in our obesogenic environment, such as fast foods, sugary drinks, a decrease in recess and physical education in schools, and more sedentary activities such as watching TV and playing computer games. What is less well known is that the prevalence of childhood obesity began to rise all across the world at approximately the same time, even in poor and undeveloped countries with little exposure to the obesogenic environment that is prominent in America.[1] Furthermore, Klimentidis et al[2] showed that 12 species of animals had an increase in body weight starting in approximately 1980 that parallels the rise in obesity in human children. This included experimental laboratory animals, domestic pets, and even rats in the sewers of Philadelphia, none of which changed their consumption of fast foods, soft drinks, or TV. These worldwide data in humans and animals suggest that simple changes in diet, lifestyle, and physical activity are not adequate to explain the rise in childhood obesity.

The rapid worldwide rise suggests that a new environmental factor appeared around 1980 that contributed to the obesity epidemic. An infectious disease could spread across the world in the pattern that has been noted, and there is an excellent candidate that should be considered: human adenovirus 36 (Adv36; Figure 10-1).[3] Adv36 was first isolated in 1978 and is different from the other 50+ human adenoviruses because the antibodies it produces do not cross-react with any of the other adenoviruses, nor do their antibodies cross-react with Adv36. This is just what might be expected in an animal virus that mutated to be able to infect humans. Scientists speculate that

Huang JS, ed. *Curbside Consultation in*
Pediatric Obesity: 49 Clinical Questions (pp 39-43).
© 2014 Taylor & Francis Group

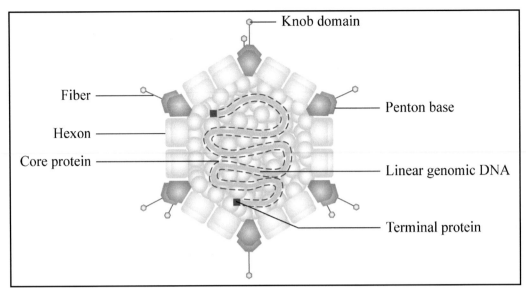

Figure 10-1. Structure of an adenovirus. (Reprinted with permission of David Darling, http://www.david-darling.info/.)

a chicken adenovirus, SMAM-1, discovered in India in the late 1970s, might be the parent virus because SMAM-1 causes obesity in chickens; one paper showed that a small number of humans appeared to have been infected with SMAM-1.[3,4]

Adv36 causes obesity by acting directly on fat cells.[5] It is a common cold virus spread by coughing and sneezing and by the fecal-oral route.[3] The initial virus infection is in the cells of the upper respiratory tract, but as the virus replicates in these cells, they die and release virus particles in the bloodstream to infect cells in all organs of the body. The Adv36 DNA gets into the nucleus of all of these cells, particularly fat cells, and turns on a number of enzymes and transcription factors that produce obesity.[6] Adv36 stimulates pathways to increase glucose transporters in the cell membrane, so more glucose gets in and the virus increases fatty acid synthase to make fatty acids out of this glucose, which increases the intracellular fat mass.[7] Other transcription factors turn on the peroxisome proliferator-activated receptor gamma pathway, which results in more fat cells being formed by differentiation from the adult stem cells in adipose tissue.[8] Thus, fat depots have bigger fat cells and more of them.

Experimental infection of animals with Adv36 shows that this virus causes increased body fat content. Chickens, mice, rats, and monkeys have all been experimentally infected, usually by introducing the virus up the nose of the animals to simulate the route by which we believe humans catch it.[3,9] A high percentage of animals get fat: approximately 60% to 90% of chickens and rodents and 100% of monkeys. Body fat and/or visceral fat (intra-abdominal fat) increases by 50% to 150% depending on the species and the experiment.[3,9] Mice and monkeys stay infectious for approximately 1 to 2 months, then the live virus is gone.[3,9] Antibody production begins rapidly after infection and when the titer becomes high enough, it prevents the virus from spreading in the individual and apparently between animals and humans. To defuse the resulting question often asked by patients (ie, "Do I have to worry about catching obesity from an obese person?") these data show that by the time a person has become obese from Adv36, the virus is long gone. In this scenario, it is the lean person with a cold who is the danger! Of course, a person who is obese from another cause could still catch Adv36, but this reminds us of the importance of infectious precautions and the need for adequate and frequent handwashing to reduce the spread of infectious disease.

We can say with confidence that Adv36 causes obesity in animals because experimental infection has been performed in several labs and the finding of increased fat tissue is consistent. Ethical reasons prevent deliberately infecting humans and watching them become obese. However, several laboratory tests can determine whether a person has been infected with Adv36. First, we can assess Adv36 antibodies present in the blood. Adv36 is unique among human adenoviruses in that it does not bind to antibodies against other adenoviruses, and Adv36 antibodies do not bind to other adenoviruses. Therefore, if antibodies to Adv36 are present, the individual specifically has been infected with Adv36. Two tests in the literature assess Adv36 antibodies: serum neutralization assay and enzyme-linked immunosorbent assay (ELISA). Most studies to date have been conducted using serum neutralization, but the recently developed ELISA is more sensitive.[10,11] The Clinical Laboratory Improvement Amendments–approved ELISA is commercially available from Obetech (www.obesityvirus.com). The second method of diagnosis is polymerase chain reaction, which looks for Adv36 DNA in tissue, usually adipose tissue.[9] This is mainly a research tool in children because it requires a needle fat biopsy rather than a simple blood draw.

Multiple investigators across the world have tested people for Adv36 antibodies; the prevalence has ranged from 6% to 65% in obese humans and 4.5% to 45% in nonobese people.[10-23] In most studies, Adv36 infection correlates with increased body weight or body mass index (kg/m^2). The association with obesity is particularly strong in children, for whom 6 of 6 studies have shown the effect.[10,11,13-16] Two studies from Korea show a prevalence of approximately 30% in obese children and 14% in nonobese children.[13,14] A study from San Diego, CA, shows that 22% of obese children and 7% of nonobese children were Adv36 positive.[15] Obese children who were Adv36 positive weighed 16 kg (35 lbs) more than Adv36-negative children. A study in 1179 children from the Czech Republic showed 28% of obese children and 21% of nonobese children were infected, with strong correlations of infection and measures of obesity.[11] A Swedish study showed 29% of obese children and 20% of nonobese children were Adv36 positive.[10] This study evaluated frozen samples from children and adults and was the first to evaluate the prevalence of Adv36 over time. In 1992, the prevalence of Adv36 in lean adults was 7%, but by 2005, the prevalence had risen to 20%. The prevalence of obesity doubled in Sweden during this time.[10] These strong associations do not prove that Adv36 causes obesity in humans, but given the animal data plus these supportive data in humans, it seems likely.

A question often asked is what to do if a person tests positive for Adv36. The following are my personal opinions. No antiviral agents are currently on the market for the treatment of Adv36, so specific treatment of the virus is not possible. For children who are already obese, standard pediatric obesity treatments of reducing calorie intake and sedentary time should be instituted and consideration given for obesity drugs to reduce further weight gain. For children who test positive but are not yet obese, constant attention to more intensive lifestyle interventions is necessary, and strong consideration should be given to the use of obesity drugs if weight gain continues. Obesity drugs are only modestly effective in reducing obesity but are more effective in preventing weight gain. For the future, antiviral agents currently under study may allow infected individuals to avoid virus-induced weight gain. A vaccine to prevent Adv36 infection is under development.

Gut Microbiota and Obesity

There have been many papers in recent years on the populations of bacteria in the intestine (ie, the gut microbiota). The role of gut bacteria in producing obesity is speculative at this point, and most of the studies are in animals. The most compelling studies showing that gut bacteria cause obesity are in animals raised germ free until being infected with different types of gut bacteria.[23] Germ-free mice delivered by Caesarian delivery have less adipose tissue than mice born normally and exposed to the environment. When these germ-free mice are given normal gut bacteria, they gain weight, a disproportionate amount of which is adipose tissue. Furthermore, if the gut micro-biota implant is from an obese mouse (genetic or diet-induced obesity) compared with an implant from a normal, lean mouse, the germ-free mice that get the gut microbes from the obese animals gain more weight and adipose tissue than those getting gut microbes from the lean animals.[23]

The selection of bacteria in the intestines of different species of mice differs according to genetic factors and by the diet fed to the mice. Feeding mice a high-fat, high-sugar diet causes a change in gut microbiota, even if the mice are chosen not to get fat on this regimen. However, getting fat alters the gut microbiota as well. A number of studies have been performed, and the populations of bacteria and their ratios associated with obesity have not always been the same for unclear reasons.[23]

The few human studies available have mainly focused on the differences in gut microbiota between obese and lean people. The same variation in findings occurs between studies in humans as in animals. Several studies suggest that the population of *Bacteroides* species is decreased and the population of *Firmicutes* species is increased in obesity.[23] If an individual loses weight by dieting or obesity surgery, the populations change to become more like those of lean people. This raises the question of whether the gut bacteria pattern causes obesity or is due to obesity.

Finally, differences in gut microbiota are associated with different levels of insulin resistance.[23] Transplantation of normal gut bacteria into mice reduces the insulin resistance that is seen in obese mice. Transplantation of human gut microbiota into humans has been performed only a few times, so little can be concluded. The overall conclusion regarding gut microbiota and human obesity or other diseases is that it is an interesting area, but much more research needs to be conducted to determine whether it will have any role in changing treatment for obesity or associated metabolic diseases.

References

1. World Health Organization. *Obesity: Preventing and Managing a Global Epidemic. Report of a WHO Consultation on Obesity, 3-5 June 1997. WHO Technical Report Series, No. 894.* Geneva, Switzerland: World Health Organization; 1998.
2. Klimentidis YC, Beasley TM, Lin HY, et al. Canaries in the coal mine: a cross-species analysis of the plurality of obesity epidemics. *Proc Biol Sci.* 2011;278(1712):1626-1632.
3. Dhurandhar NV, Israel BA, Kolesar JM, Mayhew GF, Cook ME, Atkinson RL. Increased adiposity in animals due to a human virus. *Int J Obes Relat Metab Disord.* 2000;24(8):989-996.
4. Dhurandhar NV, Kulkarni PR, Ajinkya SM, Sherikar AA, Atkinson RL. Association of adenovirus infection with human obesity. *Obes Res.* 1997;5(5):464-469.
5. Vangipuram SD, Sheele J, Atkinson RL, Holland TC, Dhurandhar NV. A human adenovirus enhances preadipocyte differentiation. *Obes Res.* 2004;12(5):770-777.
6. Whigham LD, Israel BA, Atkinson RL. Adipogenic potential of multiple human adenoviruses in vivo and in vitro in animals. *Am J Physiol Regul Integr Comp Physiol.* 2006;290(1):R190-194. Epub 2005 Sep 15.
7. Pasarica M, Shin AC, Yu M, et al. Human adenovirus 36 induces adiposity, increases insulin sensitivity, and alters hypothalamic monoamines in rats. *Obesity (Silver Spring).* 2006;14(11):1905-1913.
8. Pasarica M, Mashtalir N, McAllister EJ, et al. Adipogenic human adenovirus Ad-36 induces commitment, differen-tiation, and lipid accumulation in human adipose-derived stem cells. *Stem Cells.* 2008;26(4):969-978.
9. Dhurandhar NV, Whigham LD, Abbott DH, et al. Human adenovirus Ad-36 promotes weight gain in male rhesus and marmoset monkeys. *J Nutr.* 2002;132(10):3155-3160.
10. Almgren M, Atkinson R, He J, et al. Adenovirus-36 is associated with obesity in children and adults in Sweden as determined by rapid ELISA. *PLoS One.* 2012;7(7):e41652.
11. Hainerova I, Zamrazilová H, Atkinson RL, et al. Clinical and laboratory characteristics of 1179 Czech adolescents evaluated for antibodies to human adenovirus. *Int J Obesity.* 2013 May 14. doi: 10.1038/ijo.2013.72.
12. Atkinson RL, Dhurandhar NV, Allison DB, et al. Human adenovirus-36 is associated with increased body weight and paradoxical reduction of serum lipids. *Int J Obesity.* 2005;29:281-286.
13. Atkinson RL, Lee I, Shin HJ, He J. Human adenovirus-36 antibody status is associated with obesity in children. *Int J Pediatr Obes.* 2010;5(2):157-160. Epub 2009 Jul 1.

14. Na HN, Hong YM, Kim J, Kim HK, Jo I, Nam JH. Association between human adenovirus-36 and lipid disorders in Korean schoolchildren. *Int J Obes.* 2010;34(1):89-93. Epub 2009 Oct 13.
15. Gabbert C, Donohue M, Arnold J, Schwimmer JB. Adenovirus 36 and obesity in children and adolescents. *Pediatrics.* 2010;126(4):721-726. Epub 2010 Sep 20.
16. Tosh AK, Broy-Aschenbrenner A, El Khatib J, Ge B. Adenovirus-36 antibody status & BMI comparison among obese Missouri adolescents. *Mo Med.* 2012;109(5):402-403.
17. Trovato GM, Castro A, Tonzuso A, et al. Human obesity relationship with Ad36 adenovirus and insulin resistance. *Int J Obes (Lond).* 2009;33(12):1402-1409.
18. Trovato GM, Martines GF, Garozzo A, et al. Ad36 adipogenic adenovirus in human non-alcoholic fatty liver disease. *Liver Int.* 2010;30(2):184-190. Epub 2009 Oct 13.
19. Salehian B, Forman SJ, Kandeel FR, Bruner DE, He J, Atkinson RL. Adenovirus 36 DNA in adipose tissue of patient with unusual visceral obesity. *Emerg Infect Dis.* 2010;16(5):850-852.
20. Broderick MP, Hansen CJ, Irvine M, et al. Adenovirus 36 seropositivity is strongly associated with race and gender, but not obesity, among US military personnel. *Int J Obes (Lond).* 2010;34(2):302-308. Epub 2009 Nov 10.
21. Goossens VJ, deJager SA, Grauls GE, et al. Lack of evidence for the role of human adenovirus-36 in obesity in a European cohort. *Obesity (Silver Spring).* 2011;19(1):220-221. Epub 2009 Dec 10.
22. Rubicz R, Leach CT, Kraig E, et al. Seroprevalence of 13 common pathogens in a rapidly growing U.S. minority population: Mexican Americans from San Antonio, TX. *BMC Res Notes.* 2011;4(1):433.
23. Tagliabue A, Elli M. The role of gut microbiota in human obesity: recent findings and future perspectives. *Nutr Metab Cardiovasc Dis.* 2013;23(3):160-168.

SECTION IV

PHYSICAL ACTIVITY

QUESTION 11

I OFTEN RECOMMEND INCREASED PHYSICAL ACTIVITY TO COMBAT OBESITY. WHAT ARE THE VARIOUS BENEFITS OF INCREASED PHYSICAL ACTIVITY?

Xiaofen Deng Keating, PhD and Rulan Shangguan, PhD

The prevalence of childhood obesity in the United States has tripled since 1980.[1] Strong evidence exists that childhood obesity results in adult obesity and is associated with an elevated risk for negative health consequences such as hypertension, cardiovascular disease, type 2 diabetes, development of some types of cancer, insomnia, and sleep apnea. Furthermore, obesity negatively affects children's mental health and quality of social life through low self-esteem and depression.[2] Many of these adverse health outcomes are themselves also associated with a sedentary lifestyle, which contributes to obesity. Engagement in physical activity is thus crucial to pediatric obesity prevention and treatment.

An energy imbalance between caloric intake and expenditure (favoring intake) is a primary factor in the development of obesity, although modifiers of this equation include a complex combination of antenatal, physiologic, and genetic factors. Although we can do little to modify genetic or inherent factors, physical activity is something we can do to combat obesity and modify the risk for obesity-related factors. Guidelines recommend that children engage in 60 minutes or more of developmentally appropriate and enjoyable moderate to vigorous physical activity every day.[3] However, few children engage in sufficient physical activity on a daily basis to accrue health benefits.

Regular physical activity plays a key role in weight management and control, along with appropriate nutrition. The physiological benefits of increased physical activity include much more than weight control. Children's hearts and lungs are strengthened during physical activity, building a stronger cardiovascular system and preventing heart disease. In addition, physical activity enhances blood flow, improves carbohydrate metabolism, and increases insulin sensitivity, thus reducing the risk of metabolic diseases, including metabolic syndrome and type 2 diabetes. The possibilities of developing some types of cancers (eg, colon, breast, and endometrial cancer) that

Huang JS, ed. *Curbside Consultation in Pediatric Obesity: 49 Clinical Questions* (pp 47-49).
© 2014 Taylor & Francis Group

are associated with obesity may also be reduced by increasing physical activity and cutting down body fat.[4] Regular physical activity also facilitates the body's defense systems. When children exercise, increased breathing and sweating can help flush bacteria out of the body, increased heart rate can help circulate antibodies and white blood cells faster, and body temperature is raised temporarily, which is thought to produce an environment less conducive for bacteria to grow.[5] Increased physical activity helps build and maintain healthy bones and muscles for both normal and overweight/obese children.[6] In regard to enhanced bone mineral density, it should be noted that regular resistance exercise in particular, with specific attention on intensity and frequency (eg, squatting exercises, running stairs, or jumping rope 2 or 3 times per week), stimulates bone formation. For prepubescent children, the effects of physical activity on bone development are greater when taking place at an earlier stage of growth.

In addition to the many physical health benefits that physical activity provides to children, there are also other valuable benefits for children's brain health. During physical activity, with increased blood circulation, the brain receives more blood flow with more oxygen and nutrients, just like other parts of the body. Specifically, executive control and memory are enhanced.[7] Also, well-organized and fun physical activity may lead to lower levels of stress hormones and higher levels of growth factors that promote the growth of nerve cells. Exercise triggers the release of brain-derived neurotrophic factors that enhance the growth and connection of neurons, leading to better cognitive function.

Although the major benefits of physical activity are physiological (physical and mental), children may also derive psychological benefits from physical activity. First, physical activity may be an effective way to reduce stress and improve mood through the release of norepinephrine and endorphins. Second, self-efficacy has been shown to be positively related to higher levels of physical activity. This is likely related to children feeling more comfortable, confident, and competent to perform certain motor skills or even participate in related sports as compared with children who do not exercise regularly. Within the process of engaging in physical activity, children also learn how to achieve physical goals through effort and determination, which can be transferred to other or future goals. For children who participate in group physical activities, particularly sports, the teamwork experience provides opportunities to develop social skills such as cooperation, integrity, respect, responsibility, and conflict resolution. In sports, children also have the opportunity to take on positions of leadership. Finally, increased physical activity is one of the best interventions for insomnia. Physical activity has been shown to increase the amount of time in deep sleep (stage 4 sleep) at night. The best time for children with insomnia to exercise is 5 to 6 hours before bedtime because the drop of body temperature helps with sound sleep.

Conclusion

Physical activity provides many benefits, which are depicted in Figure 11-1. As children engage in physical activity and enjoy and recognize its many benefits, they are more likely to develop habitual physical activity for a lifetime.

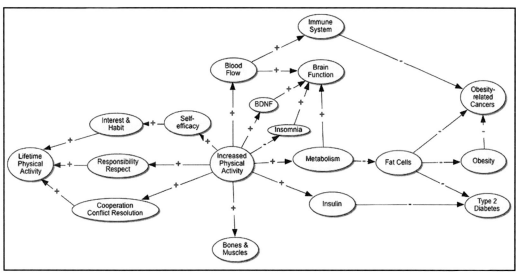

Figure 11-1. Overall benefits of increased physical activity in an obese child. BDNF = Brain-derived neurotrophic factors.

References

1. Ogden CL, Carroll MD. Prevalence of obesity among children and adolescents: United States, Trends 1963-1965 through 2007-2008. Health E-Stats. 2010. http://www.cdc.gov/nchs/data/hestat/obesity_child_07_08/obesity_child_07_08.htm. Updated June 4, 2010. Accessed March 30, 2012.
2. Griffiths LJ, Parsons TJ, Hill AJ. Self-esteem and quality of life in obese children and adolescents: a systematic review. *Int J Pediatr Obes.* 2010;5(4):282-304.
3. Strong WB, Malina RM, Blimkie CJ, et al. Evidence based physical activity for school-age youth. *J Pediatr.* 2005;146(6):732-737.
4. Warburton DE, Nicol CW, Bredin SS. Health benefits of physical activity: the evidence. *CMAJ.* 2006;174(6):801-809.
5. Pedersen BK, Hoffman-Goetz L. Exercise and the immune system: regulation, integration, and adaption. *Physiol Rev.* 2000;80(3):1055-1081.
6. US Department of Health and Human Services. *Physical Activity Guidelines Advisory Committee Report.* Washington, DC: US Department of Health and Human Services; 2008.
7. Hillman CH, Erickson KI, Kramer AF. Be smart, exercise your heart: exercise effects on brain and cognition. *Nat Rev Neurosci.* 2008;9(1):58-65.

How Do You Craft a New Exercise Regimen for Obese Children? What Is a Good Starting Point, and How Does One Advance the Program?

Brian Dauenhauer, MEd

Physical activity is any bodily movement that results in energy expenditure above basal levels. Exercise is a subset of physical activity that is structured, repetitive, and focused on improving physical fitness. Physical activity and exercise both have health benefits. When treating an obese child, general physical activity habits should be addressed first, followed by the development of a more structured exercise regimen. The treatment plan should be tailored toward the individual needs, interests, and abilities of the child and provide for maximal autonomy throughout the process. An effective program achieves not only short-term health goals, but it sets the child up for a lifetime of positive physical activity engagement.

Where to Start

When developing the physical activity component of a treatment program, a good place to start is with an evaluation of current physical activity behaviors. I recommend using a self-report instrument like the Three-Day Physical Activity Recall to estimate the child's habitual physical activity engagement and to help construct a personalized physical activity profile. Using this instrument, the child can select activities from a list and record them in 30-minute time increments for the preceding 3 days (from 7:00 AM to midnight). Intensity levels for each activity can also be recorded, ranging from light to hard. Once the report is complete, metabolic equivalent (MET) values can be assigned to each activity and summed to estimate overall energy expenditure. The resulting profile will provide an indication of when and how the child is accumulating moderate to vigorous physical activity (> 3 METs). The Centers for Disease Control and Prevention recommends children and adolescents accumulate at least 60 minutes per day.[1] This tool has been validated using accelerometry in adolescent populations,[2] but limited evidence is available to support its use with

Huang JS, ed. *Curbside Consultation in Pediatric Obesity: 49 Clinical Questions* (pp 51-54).
© 2014 Taylor & Francis Group

Table 12-1
Sample Physical Activities for Obese Children

Aerobic	Muscle Strengthening	Bone Strengthening
• A brisk walk • Playing tag • Riding a bike • Soccer, basketball, hockey • Jumping rope • Swimming	• Climbing • Yoga or Pilates • Yard work • Resistance bands • Hiking	• Jumping, hopping, leaping, balancing • Jogging • Yoga • Tennis

---

younger children. If you plan to use this tool with children under age 10 years, you should consult more closely with the child's parents to maximize accuracy.

Other measurement devices, such as pedometers and accelerometers, can also be useful in determining overall physical activity engagement (daily step-count recommendations for boys and girls are 15,000 and 12,000, respectively[3]), but one of the benefits of the guided self-report procedure is that it offers the consulting health care provider an expanded opportunity to engage with children and parents in a more in-depth conversation about some of the psychosocial factors (eg, personal interests, family culture, exercise efficacy, social support) and environmental factors (eg, community safety, access to exercise facilities, equipment) that have been recognized as important determinants of physical activity behavior. These factors should be carefully considered in developing a highly personalized treatment plan.

How to Craft a New Program

The Physical Activity Guidelines for Children and Adolescents[1] offer an appropriate overall program guide for both healthy-weight and obese children. The guidelines recommend that children aged 2 years and older participate in 60 minutes or more of physical activity on a daily basis. Participation should include aerobic activity at a moderate level most days and vigorous activity at least 3 days per week. Children should also engage in muscle- and bone-strengthening activities 3 days per week. Activities should be age appropriate, be enjoyable, and offer variety. Table 12-1 provides some sample activities that would be appropriate for obese children.

As you help design the new program, consider lifestyle physical activity first. Lifestyle physical activity can contribute substantial amounts of energy expenditure over time and thus contribute to healthy weight maintenance. Lifestyle physical activities include things like walking to and from school, riding a bike to the store, doing yard work, or cleaning the house. Depending on environmental factors like community safety, some of these activities may need adjustment. For example, certain communities have enlisted walking school buses that pair adult community members with neighborhood kids to ensure they have a safe walk to school.[4] Using the results of the physical activity self-report, try to help families identify expanded opportunities for lifestyle physical activity and see if you can address some of the obstacles that may be getting in the way. Also consider other opportunities for physical activity that may be available throughout the child's day.

In schools, children often have access to physical education classes and recess times when they are free to move their bodies. They may also attend after-school programs that allow for movement. Helping children recognize these opportunities and take advantage of them can be an effective way to build habitual physical activity into a daily routine.

Once opportunities for lifestyle physical activity have been addressed, the next step is to guide families in a critical evaluation of a child's screen time. Screen time includes watching TV, playing video games, using the computer, or messaging on a phone. Research has shown that these behaviors are related to lower levels of physical activity participation.[5] A good strategy to use with obese children is to slowly replace sedentary activities with enjoyable physical activities that have been personally selected by the child. This could mean starting with one 30-minute TV show and replacing it with outdoor play time. It could mean turning off the video game early and replacing it with a family walk. Parents should help children choose 1 or 2 times per week to begin with and then start building in more time for movement as the weeks go on. Having a list of alternative physical activities to choose from can be a useful strategy to use during this process. It is important to keep in mind that children can experience psychological dependence on certain activities like video games, so try to help families engage in the replacement process gradually and keep the decision making in the hands of the child to the greatest extent possible. As sedentary activities are gradually replaced with movement, return to the Physical Activity Guidelines to ensure that the child is being exposed to a variety of aerobic, muscle-strengthening, and bone-strengthening activities.

Advancing the Program

As new opportunities for physical activity are introduced, the FITT (frequency, intensity, time, type) principle can be used to advance the program into a more structured exercise regimen. The child can be guided in adjusting the frequency, intensity, time, or type of physical activity to progressively overload the system. For example, a family walk could be increased from 1 day a week to 3 days per week (increased frequency). Jumping rope could be progressed from single jumps to double jumps (increased intensity). Or the neighborhood bike ride could change from 2 loops to 4 (increased time). The idea is to gradually take the body out of its physiological comfort zone so that it is forced to adapt to increased demands. Children can be taught to assess their own level of exercise engagement too. They can evaluate how hard they are breathing, how fast their heart is beating, or how much they are sweating as indicators of intensity. They can report to their parents how tired they are after an activity or how sore they are the next day. It is important, however, to ensure that the progression is gradual. Children should never be in pain or feel so overwhelmed by an activity that they get hurt or risk developing an aversion. We want children to have a positive experience with exercise so that they are more likely to continue it into the future.

Once positive routines have been established, it can be helpful to guide children through a simple goal-setting process. This can help keep motivation high and encourage a greater sense of self-control. The goals can be related to any of the FITT principles mentioned previously, but should not be related to weight loss per se. Keep the focus on the process rather than the product. Also be sure that the goals are SMART (specific, measurable, attainable, realistic, timely; Figure 12-1), with an emphasis on *attainable*. We want children to experience success and build up their self-efficacy related to physical activity participation, not set them up for failure.

One final point regarding program advancement is that children should be given maximal autonomy within their plans. They should be able to choose which sedentary behaviors to limit, which physical activities to select, and how hard they wish to engage. Encouragement is welcome, but dictating a strict exercise regimen for children may be counterproductive in the long run and may lead to other types of physical and psychological harm. Concerned adults should do their best to provide a supportive and nonrestrictive physical activity environment for obese children and

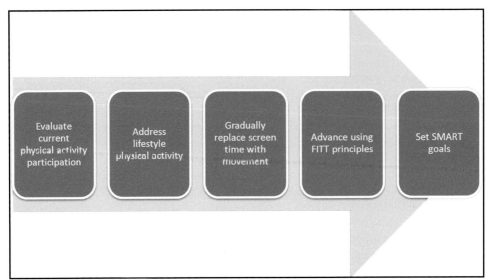

Figure 12-1. Steps in designing and advancing an exercise regimen for obese children.

facilitate the development of intrinsic motivation toward physical activity participation. A child who has positive experiences with physical activity early in life is more likely to continue engaging in it for a lifetime.

Conclusion

In designing an effective exercise program for obese children, start by evaluating a child's current physical activity participation using a self-report instrument. Use the evaluation process as an opportunity to solicit more information on some of the psychosocial and environmental factors that could influence the efficacy of the treatment. Focus first on lifestyle physical activity and try to identify ways of maximizing energy expenditure throughout a typical day. Then, using the Physical Activity Guidelines for Children and Adolescents as a guide, begin replacing screen time and other sedentary activities with more opportunities for movement. Advance the program using the FITT principles and help children set SMART goals to keep the program going strong. Throughout the process, avoid dictating a strict exercise regimen and hand over as much ownership as possible to the child. Focus not only on achieving short-term health outcomes, but also on encouraging a lifetime of healthy physical activity engagement.

References

1. US Department of Health and Human Services. *2008 Physical Activity Guidelines for Americans.* October 2008. http://www.health.gov/PAGuidelines/pdf/paguide.pdf. Accessed January 3, 2013.
2. Pate RR, Ross R, Dowda M, Trost SG, Sirard J. Validation of a three-day physical activity recall instrument in female youth. *Pediatr Exerc Sci.* 2003;15(3):257-265.
3. Tudor-Locke C, Pangrazi RP, Corbin CB, et al. BMI-referenced standards for recommended pedometer-determined steps/day in children. *Prev Med.* 2004;38(6):857-864.
4. Heelan KA, Abbey BM, Donnelly JE, Mayo MS, Welk GJ. Evaluation of a walking school bus for promoting physical activity in youth. *J Phys Act Health.* 2009;6(5):560-567.
5. Sandercock G, Ogunleye A, Voss C. Screen time and physical activity in youth: thief of time or lifestyle choice? *J Phys Act Health.* 2012;9(7):977-984.

QUESTION 13

WHEN DEVELOPING AN EXERCISE PROGRAM FOR AN OBESE CHILD, WHAT ARE THE RESTRICTIONS OR GUIDELINES TO KEEP IN MIND?

Xiaofen Deng Keating, PhD and Rulan Shangguan, PhD

Exercise programs are often prescribed for obese children to increase caloric consumption. Other benefits of physical exercise are described in Question 11. Commonly, professionals developing exercise programs for obese children look to the FITT (frequency, intensity, time, type) principles for guidance. However, existing guidelines for the exercise prescription for obese children are limited and specify only the frequency, intensity, and time of exercise needed for weight loss and prevention of weight regain, ignoring the types of exercise. Specifically, it has been suggested that obese children should engage in 150 to 300 minutes of moderate-intensity exercise weekly.[1] These guidelines do not take into account the accompanying physiological and psychosocial changes that occur with obesity, which may affect exercise performance and safety.

Physiological Considerations of Obese Children During Exercise

Increased stress on the heart (from required increased cardiac output in the setting of poor conditioning) and joints (from increased weight) and lack of balance and coordination from poor conditioning and excessive weight around the midsection may prevent obese children from engaging in certain type of exercises, such as sit-ups and push-ups. Some of the aforementioned physical limitations, however, can be adequately addressed by a conditioning, step-up exercise program that gradually increases energy expenditure and demands. Data also suggest that acute exercise or short-term exercise programs improve appetite control in the short term.[2,3]

Huang JS, ed. *Curbside Consultation in*
Pediatric Obesity: 49 Clinical Questions (pp 55-58).
© 2014 Taylor & Francis Group

INTENSITY OF EXERCISE

Vigorous exercise increases cardiac output. It has been found that the amount of stress on the heart during exercise is significantly greater in obese individuals than in people of normal weight.[4] High-intensity exercise for unconditioned obese children can severely stress the heart and cardiovascular system, putting them at a higher risk of adverse cardiac events than nonobese children. When developing exercise programs for obese children, health care professionals need to be cautious about prescribing vigorous activities at program initiation because of overbearing stress on the cardiovascular system. Instead, moderate-intensity exercise aimed to burn calories and maintain cardiovascular fitness levels are generally well tolerated and should be recommended initially.[1,5] Intensity of exercise should then be gradually increased toward levels of vigorous exercise that have been recommended (30 to 60 minutes at least 3 days per week) as part of typical weight-loss and obesity treatment regimens.[5]

TYPES OF EXERCISE

Obese children have a higher risk of fractures and knee injuries compared with children with acceptable weight.[6] In addition, obese children tend to not be as agile as nonobese children and are more likely to fall while exercising. As a result, 3 specific types of exercise should be limited or modified if possible when beginning an exercise program. First, exercise requiring excessive use of the joints should be limited. For example, jogging for approximately 30 to 60 minutes is a typical exercise for weight control and increased cardiovascular endurance. For obese children, this increases the amount of pressure on the knees and joints, which may lead to short- or long-term injuries. Similarly, weight-resistance exercises, such as squats and lunges that stress the knees and ankles, are generally not good exercise program choices for obese children. Instead, swimming and cycling may be more ideal exercises for obese children. Second, exercise requiring agility and balance, such as dodge ball, should also be limited to avoid balance disruptions and subsequent falls (in addition to accompanying embarrassment). Finally, many obese children carry weight around their midsection, which makes some exercises impossible for them to perform. For example, obese children usually have a problem performing sit-ups or push-ups because their big belly prevents them from performing it correctly. Supine exercises like push-ups can also cause problems breathing and should therefore be limited. As exercise tolerance and associated balance improve, these limitations can be removed.

EXERCISE EQUIPMENT/DEVICES

Many pieces of exercise equipment and devices are used in exercise programs and have produced excellent results. This is especially true for equipment purposed to increase strength targeting certain muscle groups. Most exercise equipment, however, is designed based on the average adult body size of the general population, with limited adjustable options. Thus, many pieces of exercise equipment are not suitable for obese children. For example, weight benches are often too narrow and/or too tall for larger bodies. Many seats on strength machines are also too small for obese children. If increasing strength in a certain region is a goal, recognize that perhaps equipment or devices may not be necessary at all and one's own body weight can be used as a form of resistance.

FOOD AS INCENTIVE

Traditionally, food (particularly sweets and candy) has been used by parents and teachers as a reward or incentive for good behaviors or achievements by children. However, with the common nutritional recommendation to limit sugar-sweetened items for obesity management, food should be avoided as an incentive for physical exercise or activity in general.

SINGLE-FACETED EXERCISE PROGRAMS

Single-faceted exercise programs target or alter only one factor at a time and should be avoided. An example of a single-faceted program might be an exercise program geared at losing weight that only increases physical activity without addressing dietary intake. These types of programs have yielded limited positive effects on obese children and should not be recommended.

Psychosocial Considerations for Exercise in Obese Children

Obese youth are at increased risk for psychosocial and psychiatric problems (see Question 27). For exercise, self-confidence and privacy can affect the success of the exercise program.

PRIVACY OF EXERCISE

Many obese children feel embarrassed to work out in public places such as gyms or public fitness facilities or in front of groups of people. In fact, it can be intimidating for an obese child to exercise in public. An exercise place that provides an adequate amount of privacy to obese children is recommended.

LOW SELF-CONFIDENCE

Obese children often have low self-confidence. Exercise programs need to help obese children build up their confidence by setting achievable goals, monitoring results, adjusting goals when needed, and celebrating goals when met.

SOCIAL AND PARENTAL SUPPORT

Social and parental support has been found to be important for children (especially girls) to adhere to exercise programs. Having parents exercise with their obese children is one of the best ways to provide support. As the age of a child increases, however, peer support plays a more important role in the success of an exercise program.

CULTURAL RELEVANCE

Cultural relevance is a relatively new but increasingly relevant concept to consider when prescribing an exercise program because the American population is more diverse than ever before. It is critical to provide children with exercises that are culturally relevant to them to increase enjoyment and buy-in, leading to increased success. For example, soccer and baseball have higher participation rates among Latino youth,[7] whereas African Americans are more likely to participate in team sports or fitness activities than their White counterparts.[8] In addition, dance can be used to improve African American and Hispanic adolescents' aerobic capacity.[9]

References

1. Daniels SR, Jacobson MS, McCrindle BW, Eckel RH, Sanner BM. American Heart Association Childhood Obesity Research Summit: executive summary. *Circulation.* 2009;119(15):2114-2123.
2. Martins C, Robertson M, Morgan LM. Effects of exercise and restrained eating behaviour on appetite control. *Proc Nutr Soc.* 2008;67(1):28-41.
3. Hagobian TA, Yamashiro M, Hinkel-Lipsker J, Streder K, Evero N, Hackney T. Effects of acute exercise on appetite hormones and ad libitum energy intake in men and women. *Appl Physiol Nutr Metab.* 2013;38(1):66-72.
4. Vella CA, Paul DR, Bader J. Cardiac response to exercise in normal-weight and obese, Hispanic men and women: implications for exercise prescription. *Acta Physiol (Oxf).* 2012;205(1):113-123.
5. Fogelholm M, Stallknecht B, Van Baak M. ECSS position statement: exercise and obesity. *Eur J Sport Sci.* 2006;6(1):15-24.
6. Stovitz SD, Pardee PE, Vazquez G, Duval S, Schwimmer JB. Musculoskeletal pain in obese children and adolescents. *Acta Paediatr.* 2008;97(4):489-493.
7. Stodolska M, Shinew KJ, Li MZ. Recreation participation patterns and physical activity among Latino visitors to three urban outdoor recreation environments. *J Park Rec Admin.* 2010;28(2):36-56.
8. Saint Onge JM, Krueger PM. Education and racial-ethnic differences in types of exercise in the United States. *J Health Soc Behav.* 2011;52(2):197-211.
9. Flores R. Dance for health: improving fitness in African American and Hispanic adolescents. *Public Health Rep.* 1995;110(2):189-193.

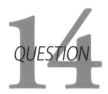

14

WHAT SOLUTIONS HAVE BEEN FOUND TO HELP CHILDREN WHO LIVE IN UNSAFE NEIGHBORHOODS OR WHO ARE HOME ALONE AND CANNOT GO OUT TO PLAY TO INCREASE THEIR PHYSICAL ACTIVITY?

Xiaofen Deng Keating, PhD and Rulan Shangguan, PhD

There are a variety of outdoor and indoor activities that children living in unsafe neighborhoods can perform to accrue the health benefits of exercise. Some of the solutions need special organization or community investment, whereas others require limited resources. The following are low-cost solutions for families with limited means.

Community Resources

USING A WALKING/BIKING-TO-SCHOOL PROGRAM

Previous research demonstrates that children who walk to school are less likely to become obese.[1] In unsafe neighborhoods, walks with children should be supervised by parents, school staff, and local volunteers. Factors such as the distance to school and local weather conditions may affect the availability of such programs.

ATTENDING AN AFTER-SCHOOL EXERCISE PROGRAM

After-school exercise or health promotion programs have been widely implemented in school settings, especially in high-risk areas.[2-4] Unfortunately, attendance remains low because many parents are unaware of the availability of such programs, do not know how to choose a good after-school program, or have yet to recognize the importance of increasing their children's engagement in exercise. Although it remains unclear which after-school program elements can generate the

Huang JS, ed. *Curbside Consultation in Pediatric Obesity: 49 Clinical Questions* (pp 59-61).
© 2014 Taylor & Francis Group

best effects on promoting exercise among obese youth, the following are general attributes for ideal after-school programs[4] that can be used as guidance for selecting an after-school program:

- Adequate facilities and equipment to allow variety and choice in physical activities
- A flexible and relaxed schedule
- A safe environment
- Opportunities to explore ideas, feelings, and identities
- Avenues for self-expression, such as exploration of one's own heritage
- Scheduled time for unstructured play and simple fun
- Free and flexible transportation support

Indoor Activities

INCORPORATING HOUSEWORK INTO THE DAILY EXERCISE ROUTINE

It will depend on the age of the child, but housecleaning, grocery shopping, cooking, and washing dishes by hand may be used as forms of exercise. Wherever and whenever age appropriate, children should be asked to help out with these tasks. This strategy also has a wonderful by-product—increased quality time among family members.

INVITING OTHER KIDS TO COME HOME TO PLAY

Play is fundamental to a child's physical and psychological development. Although the concept of play is broad, "play" here refers to specific child play with appropriate materials/equipment and environments that produce quality physical activity. For instance, many children, especially younger ones, play hide and seek at home. If parents set up the environment to allow for limited running (ie, unobstructed by furniture or other home hazards) and/or stair climbing, children can gain a great deal of exercise.

USING STAIRS TO ENGAGE IN AEROBIC EXERCISE

Home or apartment stairs can be effectively used as a good place for exercise. Spending 30 minutes to 1 hour walking, jogging, or hopping up and down the stairs can be a great workout and can burn serious calories.

JOGGING IN PLACE

For children whose homes do not have stairs, jogging in place can get the heart rate up. An obese child may want to try multiple 5- to 10-minute intervals with short breaks in between or go for a full 30 minutes, depending on their level of exercise tolerance and conditioning. It is important to point out that jogging in place is repetitive and boring. It might help to play accompanying music for children to listen to while jogging in place.

JUMPING ROPE

Jumping rope is a simple activity, but it requires substantial energy to perform. It is a great way to get an aerobic workout and get a child's heart pumping. It is also great for the legs and calves and hand-eye coordination. An obese child can work up a good sweat after jumping rope for even just 10 to 15 minutes.

EXERCISE CREATED BY MODERN TECHNOLOGY

Technology can be used as a great alternative for homebound children to increase exercise and can be implemented to varying degrees based on financial resources. One type of exercise can be accomplished by using videos. Although it requires money to buy the video and exercise equipment, which can be expensive, many families, even with limited resources, still have access to a television and DVD player. Exercise DVDs are available from most public libraries for free. In fact, various workout videos are available, ranging from low-intensity workouts for beginners to high-intensity workouts for advanced exercisers. These DVDs can provide an easy way to have a directed at-home workout. More important, most children find it fun. For those with more financial resources available, gaming systems such as the Nintendo Wii, Dance Dance Revolution (Konami Corporation), and exergaming can provide great exercise programs for homebound children. Pilates is another great at-home workout. Again, it may require the use of an instructional DVD at first or a quick Google search for a YouTube video, but it can be a great way to stay fit.

Conclusion

Children living in unsafe neighborhoods have some restrictions to outdoor exercise places/facilities. However, it is still possible to obtain an adequate amount of exercise to accrue the health benefits of exercise by engaging in physically active indoor activities and/or by incorporating physical activity into the daily routine. Overall, children can gain enough exercise by performing housework, grocery shopping, walking or biking to school in groups with the supervision of adults, joining an after-school exercise program, and playing with friends at home. Furthermore, modern technologies have opened new possibilities for indoor exercise, which can be both fun and intensive at the same time.

References

1. Mori N, Armada F, Willcox DC. Walking to school in Japan and childhood obesity prevention: new lessons from an old policy. *Am J Pub Health.* 2012;102(11):2068-2073.
2. Stice E, Shaw H, Marti CN. A meta-analytic review of prevention programs for children and adolescents: the skinny on interventions that work. *Psychol Bull.* 2006;132(5):667-691.
3. Daud R, Carruthers C. Outcome study of an after-school program for youth in a high-risk environment. *J Park Rec Admin.* 2008;26(2):95-114.
4. Halpern R. After-school programs for low-income children: promise and challenges. *Future Child.* 1999;9(2):81-95.

SECTION V

COMORBIDITIES

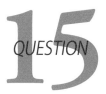

WHAT MALNUTRITION ISSUES SHOULD I CONSIDER IN THE OBESE CHILD?

Denise Purdie, MD and Mary Abigail S. Garcia, MD

For most Western physicians, the terms *undernutrition* or *malnutrition* conjure images of children in developing countries with protein-calorie malnutrition: the skinny limbs and protuberant bellies of kwashiorkor or the wasted-away appearance of marasmus. However, obese children can also be considered undernourished in terms of certain vitamins and minerals. Technically, the obese child consumes sufficient calories to meet, and more often exceed, his or her daily energy requirements. However, his or her diet is fundamentally lacking in unprocessed nutrient-rich foods such as fresh fruits, vegetables, and whole grains, which puts him or her at risk for developing micronutrient deficiencies. Therefore, his or her nutritional intake is essentially unbalanced.

Macronutrients include carbohydrates, fats, and proteins, which are responsible for energy intake in a child's diet. The obese child—like most healthy children in the United States—is not at risk for protein-calorie malnutrition because he or she consumes at least the minimum calories and proteins recommended on a daily basis.

However, the obese child is at risk for multiple micronutrient deficiencies. Micronutrients include vitamins, minerals, and trace elements. Children are already more susceptible to deficiencies in these nutrients because of increased requirements during the rapid growth experienced in infancy and adolescence. Micronutrient deficiencies can unfortunately be common in the case of the obese child, who is more likely to eat high-calorie processed foods or junk foods that are low in nutritional quality. Specific deficiencies are described in the upcoming pages.

Huang JS, ed. *Curbside Consultation in
Pediatric Obesity: 49 Clinical Questions* (pp 65-68).
© 2014 Taylor & Francis Group

Vitamins

Multiple studies have shown the obese child and adult to be deficient in vitamins D, E, and A.[1] There has been some thought that low circulating levels of these fat-soluble vitamins might be related to increased storage in excess adipose tissue in addition to decreased intake.

You are likely aware of the increasing prevalence of vitamin D insufficiency and deficiency in the pediatric population. Vitamin D is important in maintaining serum calcium and phosphorus concentrations; in addition, it has recently been linked to cardiovascular health and cancer prevention. Dietary intake of vitamin D comes primarily from fortified milk products and cereals, but sunlight exposure is also an important source. Vitamin D is also present naturally in some foods such as fatty fish and seal liver, but you are unlikely to find a child in the contiguous Unites States eating these. Deficiency in the obese child is thought to be the result of multiple factors, including decreased intake of fortified milk products because of increased consumption of sweetened beverages (such as juice or soda). In addition, the more sedentary lifestyle of the obese child often leads to decreased exposure to sunlight, which has been thought to contribute to the development of hypovitaminosis D. Evaluating for vitamin D deficiency should include a serum 25-hydroxyvitamin D level rather than 1,25-hydroxyvitamin D. The former, the circulating form of vitamin D, is a more accurate reflection of vitamin D status. In addition to supplementation with vitamin D for those found deficient, calcium intake should at least meet dietary reference index for age. Otherwise, calcium supplementation should also be provided for optimal bone health.

Vegetable oil, unprocessed cereal grains, nuts, fruits, and vegetables are sources of vitamin E (alpha-tocopherol), which is important in preventing damage related to oxidative stress. This vitamin is destroyed during the processing of packaged and processed foods. Vitamin A (retinol and beta-carotene) is found in liver, fish, dairy products, dark-colored fruit, and leafy vegetables. It is required for normal vision, gene expression, embryonic development, and immune function. Because of poor intake of vitamin E– and vitamin A–rich foods, the obese child is at risk for these deficiencies. Serum alpha-tocopherol levels are altered by cholesterol and triglyceride levels. Increased levels of serum lipids will falsely lower alpha-tocopherol levels; therefore, cholesterol and triglyceride levels should be obtained when screening for vitamin E deficiency. Vitamin A status can be determined by measuring either serum retinol or serum carotene levels, although these do not always reflect total body stores. For example, serum retinol levels reflect the amount of vitamin bound to retinol binding protein, which can be affected by malnutrition and infection.

In addition, the obese child has been shown to be at risk for deficiency in certain B vitamins, such as cobalamin and thiamine. Fortified cereals, meat, fish, and poultry are rich in vitamin B12, which is a coenzyme in nucleic acid metabolism and necessary for the production of hemoglobin. Deficiency has been associated with various hematologic, neurologic, and psychiatric disorders, such as megaloblastic anemia, peripheral neuropathy, dementia, and depression. A variety of methods are used to measure cobalamin levels, including chemiluminescence and radioassay methods. Therefore, it is important to consider levels with a specific laboratory's reference range in mind. In addition, there are limitations in the accuracy of measuring a single cobalamin level because of high intratesting variability and low positive predictive value. If the clinical picture is suspicious for vitamin B12 deficiency (ie, macrocytic anemia), consider an empiric trial of therapy.

Enriched, fortified, or whole-grain products are the main source of thiamine, although it is also abundant in yeast, beef, pork, and legumes. Refined carbohydrates, which are central to the obese child's diet, have minimal amounts of this mineral. Thiamine is a coenzyme in carbohydrate and branched-chain amino acid metabolism and are therefore important in tissue and organ function. Deficiency occurs quickly because large quantities are not stored in tissue, and it has been associated with cardiovascular and neurologic dysfunction (eg, wet and dry beriberi, Wernicke-Korsakoff syndrome). Thiamine deficiency should be evaluated by measuring the serum thiamine concentration.

Interestingly, folic acid or folate—another water-soluble B vitamin—has not been shown to be deficient in the obese individual.[1] This is likely because of the fortification of common foods, especially cereals, with folic acid per United States Food and Drug Administration regulations.

Minerals

Despite the number of cereals and breads fortified with minerals, the obese child appears to be at risk for deficiencies in iron, zinc, selenium, and magnesium.[2]

Iron is a critical component of multiple enzymes, cytochromes, myoglobin, and hemoglobin. Heme sources of iron include meat, poultry, and fish, whereas nonheme sources include dairy, eggs, fortified breads, and cereals. Iron deficiency results in anemia and has been associated with decreased alertness and impaired learning in children. Some studies have suggested that, given the negative correlation of serum iron levels and body mass index, obese children should be routinely screened for iron deficiency anemia.[2] The mechanism for iron deficiency in obese patients is not fully elucidated but is likely to be associated with decreased absorption related to increased adipose-induced inflammation.[3]

Zinc's role as a catalyst for hundreds of enzymes makes it essential for proper growth and development. It is important for immune function and wound healing. Dietary sources of zinc include meats, shellfish, legumes, fortified breads, and cereals. Deficiency leads to decreased growth, acrodermatitis enteropathica (diarrhea with dermatitis around orifices), impaired immunity, and poor wound healing. Generally, serum zinc levels are reflective of total stores; however, they can be falsely decreased by acute or chronic inflammation or hypoalbuminemia. Serum alkaline phosphatase can also provide a clue because zinc deficiency results in low alkaline phosphatase levels. Indirect markers such as serum superoxide dismutase or erythrocyte alkaline phosphatase activity are not widely available.

Selenium is a trace element that is found mostly in plants, especially vegetables grown in areas with high selenium content in the soil. It can also be found in meat, seafood, whole grains, and garlic. Selenium is incorporated into protein to make selenoproteins. Selenoproteins are important in preventing oxidative damage and regulating thyroid and immune function. Deficiency can produce cardiomyopathy, hypothyroidism, and immune dysfunction.

Dietary magnesium is found mostly in dark leafy vegetables, although legumes, spices, coffee, tea, fish, soy, nuts, and whole grains also serve as sources of this mineral. Magnesium is required for the function of hundreds of enzymes, including all enzymes using or synthesizing adenosine triphosphate. Neuromuscular and myocardial activity also rely on magnesium. Overt deficiency is relatively rare; however, anorexia, nausea, vomiting, fatigue, and weakness can be seen in early deficiency. Numbness, tingling, muscle cramps, seizures, and arrhythmias can occur as levels further decrease.

The reasons for these mineral deficiencies in the obese child are not fully understood but are likely at least partly due to diets that are unbalanced and unhealthy.

Complications

Most obese patients do not show overt symptoms of malnutrition despite mild deficiencies seen in their serum levels. The extremes of vitamin and mineral deficiencies described previously are rarely seen in the pre- or postoperative obese child. However, pediatricians and other medical providers must be aware that caution should be taken, especially with those patients who are undergoing bariatric surgery. Food intake and/or food absorption decrease significantly in the postoperative period; thus, patients are at a further increased risk of major nutrient deficiencies if not fully repleted preoperatively and supplemented postoperatively. In contrast to the preoperative period, there have been cases of kwashiorkor, microcytic anemia, acrodermatitis enteropathica, and neurologic dysfunction in patients after bariatric surgery.[4]

In addition, deficiencies of multiple micronutrients have been associated themselves with insulin resistance, impaired glucose metabolism, hypertension, hyperlipidemia, and immune dysfunction, which are traditionally considered the consequences of obesity. For example, zinc regulates leptin secretion and promotes glucose uptake in adipose tissue. The synthesis and action of insulin also hinges on the activity of zinc. It should come as no surprise that studies have related low levels of zinc with the metabolic syndrome as well as diabetes mellitus.[2] Low magnesium levels have also been associated with insulin resistance in children, along with hypertension and hyperlipidemia.[2]

Lower bone density and fractures have been associated with obesity in children. Prepubertal bone fractures and later development of osteoporosis may result from inadequate calcium and vitamin D.

Recommendations

The malnutrition issues of the obese child might be thought of as *famine in the midst of plenty*. Despite an abundance of available foods, the obese child's diet lacks important micronutrients. Although there are no official recommendations to regularly obtain levels of micronutrients in obese children, a thorough dietary assessment to estimate daily intake of macronutrients and micronutrients should be performed. The obese child's intake should be compared with the recommended dietary reference intake established by the Food and Nutrition Board of the Institute of Medicine. The *American Academy of Pediatrics Nutrition Handbook* is another reliable source of appropriate caloric, macronutrient, and micronutrient intakes at various ages. Although this is important in all obese children, it is imperative that micronutrient monitoring and supplementation occur in adolescent patients considering gastric bypass surgery—both before and after the procedure.

However, the solution should not be to simply add supplements but to educate the obese child and his or her family about healthy, balanced nutrition. Both the American Heart Association and American Academy of Pediatrics recommend that individuals older than 2 years consume a diet rich in fruits, vegetables, whole grains, low-fat and nonfat dairy products, beans, fish, and lean meat. The American Heart Association has provided implementation strategies for their dietary guidelines to help the general pediatrician.[5] Regular physical activity is also an important component of these recommendations, which will not only increase exposure to sunlight (and vitamin D) but also decrease adiposity and increase muscle mass. You (and your patient) will have the best chance at success with frequent monitoring and family involvement.

References

1. Kaidar-Person O, Person B, Szomstein S, Rosenthal RJ. Nutritional deficiencies in morbidly obese patients: a new form of malnutrition? Part A: vitamins. *Obes Surg.* 2008;18(7):870-876.
2. Kaidar-Person O, Person B, Szomstein S, Rosenthal RJ. Nutritional deficiencies in morbidly obese patients: a new form of malnutrition? Part B: minerals. *Obes Surg.* 2008;18(8):1028-1034.
3. McClung JP, Karl JP. Iron deficiency and obesity: the contribution of inflammation and diminished iron absorption. *Nutr Rev.* 2008;67(2):100-104.
4. Xanthakos SA. Nutritional deficiencies in obesity and after bariatric surgery. *Pediatric Clin N Am.* 2009;56(5):1105-1121.
5. Gidding SS, Dennison BA, Birch LL, et al. Dietary recommendations for children and adolescents: a guide for practitioners. *Pediatrics.* 2006;117(2):544-559.

16
QUESTION

WHAT ARE THE COMMON GASTROINTESTINAL DISEASES ASSOCIATED WITH CHILDHOOD OBESITY?

Lillian J. Choi, MD and Kimberly Montez, MD

Obesity is now a prevalent childhood epidemic that is associated with a number of gastrointestinal (GI) issues. GI symptoms associated with obesity are nevertheless not specific to obese patients and can be seen across all ages and weight categories and along with other disorders. Effective management of the obese patient presenting with GI complaints begins with recognizing the role of obesity in the development of the GI disorder and thus requires the addressing of both the obesity and its associated comorbidity.

The GI disorders associated with childhood obesity that will be discussed here include gastroesophageal reflux disease (GERD), cholelithiasis and its related complications, and functional GI disorders (FGIDs; Table 16-1). It is important to briefly mention the silent GI complications of obesity, nonalcoholic fatty liver disease and nonalcoholic steatohepatitis (discussed in Question 17). Left unmanaged, they can lead to liver cirrhosis and failure. This highlights the need to screen obese patients even in the absence of symptoms. Similarly, it is important to recognize that children with obesity may also have GI disorders more typically associated with weight loss or poor weight gain—in particular, celiac disease and inflammatory bowel disease.

Abdominal pain is a common complaint in pediatrics. Although the differential diagnosis of abdominal pain in pediatrics is extensive and can be daunting, appreciating the increased prevalence of certain disorders associated with abdominal pain in the obese child can provide a starting point for your evaluation.

GERD is probably the most recognized obesity-associated complication. Children with reflux will usually complain of a sharp or burning epigastric abdominal pain typically occurring shortly after meals. In addition to abdominal pain, these children will often complain of an acid or bitter taste in their mouth, regurgitation, vomiting, and substernal chest pain. You should further inquire about pulmonary symptoms because reflux can manifest as chronic cough, nocturnal cough, asthma, and pneumonia (Table 16-2).[1]

Huang JS, ed. *Curbside Consultation in Pediatric Obesity: 49 Clinical Questions* (pp 69-76).
© 2014 Taylor & Francis Group

Table 16-1

Gastrointestinal Disorders Associated With Obesity

Esophagus
- Gastroesophageal reflux disease

Biliary System
- Cholelithiasis
- Cholecystitis
- Choledocholithiasis
- Cholangitis
- Biliary pancreatitis

Functional Gastrointestinal Disorders
- Constipation and encopresis
- Functional abdominal pain
- Functional dyspepsia
- Irritable bowel syndrome

Liver
- Nonalcoholic fatty liver disease
- Nonalcoholic steatohepatitis

Table 16-2

Gastroesophageal Reflux Disease[1]

Common Symptoms	*Pulmonary Symptoms*	*Warning Symptoms*
• Acid taste in mouth • Nausea • Regurgitation • Emesis • Abdominal pain-epigastric • Substernal chest pain	• Chronic cough • Nocturnal cough • Asthma • Pneumonia	• Hematemesis • Treatment failure • Relapse of symptoms after stopping treatment

Table 16-3
Biliary Tract Disorders: Signs, Symptoms and Evaluation

	Cholelithiasis	*Cholecystitis*	*Biliary Pancreatitis*
Signs/symptoms	• Biliary colic • Abdominal pain-epigastric or right upper quadrant • Nausea • Emesis • Jaundice • Intolerance to fatty foods • (–) Murphy's sign	• Abdominal pain—severe persistent epigastric or right upper quadrant • Nausea • Emesis • Fever • (+) Murphy's sign	• Abdominal pain—epigastric or upper quadrant pain that may radiate to the back • Nausea • Emesis • Anorexia
Laboratory evaluation	• Normal	• Leukocytosis	• Elevated amylase and lipase (3 times upper limit of normal)
Abdominal ultrasonography	• Echogenic stones in the gallbladder	• Gallbladder wall thickening • Gallbladder wall dilation • Pericholecystic fluid • Sonographic Murphy's sign	• Choledocho-lithiasis • Extensive sludge in gallbladder • Pancreas may appear edematous and hypoechoic

Although the pathophysiology is not completely understood, abdominal obesity increasing intragastric pressure and gastroesophageal pressure gradient, increased frequency of transient lower esophageal sphincter relaxations, and/or formation of a hiatal hernia have been implicated as potential mechanisms in GERD associated with obesity.[2] The North American Society of Pediatric Gastroenterology, Hepatology and Nutrition (NASPGHAN) 2009 GERD guidelines support empiric treatment of older children and adolescents with symptoms or signs of GERD with a proton pump inhibitor for up to 4 weeks. It is important to realize, however, that although therapy may provide symptom relief or resolution, this is not diagnostic of GERD. There is no evidence to support empirically treating infants or young children for GERD.[1] However, if the child has severe or persistent symptoms, hematemesis, or dysphagia; fails treatment; or relapses after completing therapy, the child should be referred to a gastroenterologist as these symptoms may warrant further endoscopic evaluation to assess for other causes such as erosive esophagitis and eosinophilic esophagitis (see Table 16-2).

If your obese patient describes recurrent colicky pain in the right upper quadrant (RUQ) or epigastric area, consider disorders of the biliary tract (Table 16-3). Obesity is a well-established risk factor for cholelithiasis in adults and is becoming increasingly recognized as a risk factor for gallstones in children. The risk of cholesterol-type gallstones increases with increasing body mass index (which may reflect an unhealthy diet composition) and is greater in females than males, with this risk further increasing in females who take oral contraceptives.[3,4] Cholelithiasis can be asymptomatic or it can present with biliary colic, epigastric, or RUQ pain, nausea, emesis, jaundice, and intolerance to food, particularly fatty food. The physical examination and laboratory evaluations are generally benign.

If the obese child develops more severe or persistent epigastric/RUQ abdominal pain that is associated with fever, nausea, and/or vomiting, consider evaluating for complications of cholelithiasis: cholecystitis, cholangitis, or biliary pancreatitis. Cholecystitis, inflammation of the gallbladder, results when a gallstone obstructs the cystic duct, and biliary pancreatitis results when a gallstone traverses the common bile duct, lodges at the sphincter of Oddi, and obstructs the pancreatic duct. Cholangitis is infection of the common bile duct. Patients with these complications may appear jaundiced. Characteristic symptoms of biliary pancreatitis include abdominal pain that radiates to the back and anorexia.

On physical examination of the abdomen in the child whom you suspect has biliary tract issues, you should evaluate for Murphy's sign. Murphy's sign is defined as the arrest of inspiration due to pain when the gallbladder is palpated at the RUQ and is the sign classically associated with cholecystitis. Evaluation of cholelithiasis and its complications should also include laboratory studies (a comprehensive metabolic panel, complete blood counts with differential, pancreatic enzymes, and fasting lipid panel) and an abdominal sonography, which is the diagnostic imaging of choice for evaluation of cholelithiasis. It is important to instruct your patient to fast for 8 hours prior to the study because this allows for gallbladder relaxation and distention, which allows for better visualization of the echogenic gallstones. Table 16-3 reviews the common findings associated with these disorders.

Patients with cholecystitis, cholangitis, or biliary pancreatitis require admission to the hospital for management. This includes intravenous hydration, bowel rest, intravenous antibiotics for cholecystitis and cholangitis, pain management, and surgical consultation. Most of these patients will eventually require cholecystectomy. In patients with uncomplicated cholelithiasis, dietary modification (a low-fat diet) is an essential element of therapy. As previously mentioned, a fasting lipid panel is an important part of the evaluation in an obese child with cholelithiasis because cholelithiasis may be indicative of dyslipidemia.

Unlike GERD and cholelithiasis, in which the association with obesity has been well established, data regarding the association of obesity with the FGIDs are less clear. This group of disorders, which includes functional constipation and encopresis, functional abdominal pain, functional dyspepsia, and irritable bowel syndrome, will therefore be briefly discussed here.

The FGIDs can be frustrating in regard to diagnosis and management for both the practitioner and the patient and family. These disorders are characterized by persistence of GI symptoms without evidence of any physiologic, anatomic, or biochemical abnormalities. The ROME III criteria for the aforementioned FGIDs are presented in Tables 16-4 through 16-7 and serve as guidelines for diagnosing these FGIDs.[5-7]

The mechanism by which obesity is associated with functional abdominal pain is likely multifactorial. In particular, it has been hypothesized that lack of exercise and poor diet, one that is higher in saturated fats and lower in fiber-rich foods such as fruits and vegetables, may play a role in functional constipation and functional abdominal pain.[8] Furthermore, dysregulation between the central nervous system and enteric nervous system, known as the *brain-gut axis*, has also been implicated as having a role in the pathophysiology of functional abdominal pain that results in visceral hyperalgesia.[5]

Table 16-4
Rome III Criteria for the Diagnosis of Functional Constipation in Children Aged 4 to 18 Years[7]

At Least 2 of the Following Present for ≥ 2 Months
- Two or fewer defecations per week
- At least one episode of incontinence per week
- History of retentive posturing or excessive volitional stool retention
- History of painful or hard bowel movements
- Presence of a large fecal mass in the rectum
- History of large-diameter stools that may obstruct the toilet

Reprinted from *Gastroenterology*, 130(5), Rasquin A, Di Lorenzo C, Forbes D, et al, Childhood functional gastrointestinal disorders: child/adolescent, 1527-1537, Copyright 2006 with permission from Elsevier.

Table 16-5
Rome III Criteria for the Diagnosis of Functional Abdominal Pain in Children Aged 4 to 18 Years[7]

Within the Preceding 2 Months, at Least Weekly Occurrence of (Must Include All of the Following Symptoms):
- Episodic or continuous abdominal pain, **and**
- Insufficient criteria for other gastrointestinal disorders, **and**
- No evidence of inflammatory, anatomic, metabolic, or neoplastic process to explain symptoms

Reprinted from *Gastroenterology*, 130(5), Rasquin A, Di Lorenzo C, Forbes D, et al, Childhood functional gastrointestinal disorders: child/adolescent, 1527-1537, Copyright 2006 with permission from Elsevier.

When considering FGIDs, your evaluation should start with a thorough history and physical examination, including pelvic, genitourinary, and rectal examination, being attentive to any alarm signs or symptoms (Table 16-8).

The presence of any alarm symptoms or signs warrants further evaluation for other organic causes. Fecal occult blood test to evaluate for a potential organic etiology has also been recommended by the NASPGHAN. Depending on your history and physical examination, you may consider additional laboratory or imaging studies. However, you should recognize that one

Table 16-6

Rome III Criteria for the Diagnosis of Functional Dyspepsia in Children Aged 4 to 18 Years[7]

Within the Preceding 2 Months, At Least Weekly Occurrence of (Must Include All of the Following Symptoms):
- Persistent or recurring pain or discomfort in the upper abdomen, **and**
- No evidence of inflammatory, anatomic, metabolic, or neoplastic process to explain symptoms, **and**
- Pain or discomfort not relieved by defecation or associated with the onset of a change in stool frequency or form

Reprinted from *Gastroenterology*, 130(5), Rasquin A, Di Lorenzo C, Forbes D, et al, Childhood functional gastrointestinal disorders: child/adolescent, 1527-1537, Copyright 2006 with permission from Elsevier.

Table 16-7

Rome III Criteria for the Diagnosis of Irritable Bowel Syndrome in Children Aged 4 to 18 Years[7]

Within the Preceding 2 Months, At Least Weekly Occurrence of (Must Include All of the Following Symptoms):
- Abdominal discomfort or pain associated with at least 2 of the following:
  - Relieved with defecation, **and/or**
  - Onset associated with a change in frequency of stool, **and/or**
  - Onset associated with a change in form of stool, **and**
- No evidence of inflammatory, anatomic, metabolic, or neoplastic process to explain symptoms

Reprinted from *Gastroenterology*, 130(5), Rasquin A, Di Lorenzo C, Forbes D, et al, Childhood functional gastrointestinal disorders: child/adolescent, 1527-1537, Copyright 2006 with permission from Elsevier.

approach to reducing patient anxiety and dissatisfaction during the evaluation for FGIDs (usually resulting from extensive testing of patients with negative results) is to minimize testing in patients who do not have alarm signs or symptoms. If there are any concerns or alarm signs or symptoms, patients should be referred to gastroenterology for further evaluation. Referral to the subspecialist for management of FGIDs may also be appropriate in the setting of persistent or severe symptoms

Table 16-8
Warning Symptoms and Signs in a Child With Abdominal Pain[5,7]

Symptoms	*Signs*
• Weight loss • Deceleration of linear growth • Gastrointestinal bleed • Significant vomiting • Chronic diarrhea • Persistent RUQ or right lower quadrant abdominal pain • Unexplained fever	• Localized RUQ or right lower quadrant abdominal pain • Hepatomegaly • Splenomegaly • Localized fullness or mass on abdominal examination • Costovertebral angle tenderness • Spinal tenderness • Perianal abnormalities
• Family history of inflammatory bowel disease	

Reprinted from *Gastroenterology*, 130(5), Rasquin A, Di Lorenzo C, Forbes D, et al, Childhood functional gastrointestinal disorders: child/adolescent, 1527-1537, Copyright 2006 with permission from Elsevier.

because treatment of such symptoms often must be individualized and often requires a multifaceted approach inclusive of the gastroenterologist, counseling, and biofeedback.

Conclusion

With the rising incidence of obesity in children, we are now seeing an increasing prevalence of GI issues related to this growing problem. We hope that increased understanding and awareness of these comorbidities will translate into improved assessment, family and patient education, prevention, and overall management of GI issues in the obese child. Considering the underlying risk for the previously mentioned GI comorbidities, it is imperative to address the child's weight and incorporate education on healthy lifestyle choices as a vital part of the management of any GI issue in the obese child.

References

1. Vandenplas Y, Rudolph CD, Di Lorenzo C, et al. Pediatric gastroesophageal reflux clinical practice guidelines: joint recommendations of the North American Society for Pediatric Gastroenterology, Hepatology, and Nutrition (NASPGHAN) and the European Society for Pediatric Gastroenterology, Hepatology, and Nutrition (ESPGHAN). *J Pediatr Gastroenterol Nutr.* 2009;49(4):498-547.
2. Teitelbaum JE, Sinha P, Micale M, Yeung S, Jaeger J. Obesity is related to multiple functional abdominal diseases. *J Pediatr.* 2009;154(3):444-446.

3. Koebnick C, Smith N, Black MH, et al. Pediatric obesity and gallstone disease. *J Pediatr Gastroenterol Nutr.* 2012;55(3):328-333.
4. Poffenberger CM, Gausche-Hill M, Ngai S, Myers A, Andrew BS, Renslo R. Cholelithiasis and its complications in children and adolescents: update and case discussion. *Pediatr Emerg Care.* 2012;28(1):68-76.
5. American Academy of Pediatrics Subcommittee on Chronic Abdominal Pain. Chronic abdominal pain in children. *Pediatrics.* 2005;115(3):812-815.
6. Pashankar DS, Loening-Baucke V. Increased prevalence of obesity in children with functional constipation evaluated in an academic medical center. *Pediatrics.* 2005;116(3):e377-e380.
7. Rasquin A, Di Lorenzo C, Forbes D, et al. Childhood functional gastrointestinal disorders: child/adolescent. *Gastroenterology.* 2006;130(5):1527-1537.
8. Malaty HM, Abudayyeh S, Fraley K, Graham D, Gilger MA, Hollier DR. Recurrent abdominal pain in school children: effect of obesity and diet. *Acta Pediatr.* 2007;96(4):572-576.

WHAT SHOULD I DO WITH AN OBESE CHILD WHO HAS AN ELEVATED LIVER FUNCTION TEST?

Kimberly P. Newton, MD and Jeffrey B. Schwimmer, MD

Obese children are at an increased risk for nonalcoholic fatty liver disease (NAFLD).[1] The American Academy of Pediatrics recommends that overweight and obese children be screened for NAFLD using serum alanine aminotransferase (ALT) and aspartate aminotransferase (AST).[2] Prevalence of elevated ALT in obese children ranges from 10% to 25%.[3] If children are screened according to guidelines, many will have abnormal results. Interpreting these results and acting accordingly is a complicated process. One must determine the degree and nature of liver enzyme abnormality, whether there is an urgent problem requiring prompt referral to a specialist, and the etiology of the abnormality because not all liver enzyme elevation is due to NAFLD.

Elevated ALT and AST activity commonly serve as markers of hepatocellular injury and necrosis. ALT and AST are both highly concentrated in the liver, but AST is also significantly present in the heart, skeletal muscle, brain, kidneys, and red blood cells; therefore, ALT is regarded as more liver specific. When confronted with ALT and AST measurements in an obese child, the primary care provider must first determine whether results are normal or abnormal. The reference ranges provided for laboratory interpretation are often generated by analyses of poorly characterized local populations and thus may not be truly normal, including individuals with unrecognized disease. The Screening ALT For Elevation in Today's Youth study was performed to develop a more accurate, biology-based normal of ALT for the pediatric population.[4] Biology-based reference ranges for ALT were determined among a large population-based sample of children after excluding individuals with hepatotoxic medication exposure, possible NAFLD, hepatitis B virus, hepatitis C virus, human immunodeficiency virus (HIV), and iron overload. The 95th percentile of ALT was found to be 25.8 U/L for boys and 22.1 U/L for girls, which is much lower than 53 U/L—the median upper limit of normal ALT at children's hospitals nationwide. Thus, a laboratory value of 52 U/L that is considered within the normal reference range for boys at many

Huang JS, ed. *Curbside Consultation in
Pediatric Obesity: 49 Clinical Questions* (pp 77-82).
© 2014 Taylor & Francis Group

hospitals would be 2 times the upper limit of normal of the biology-based value. As such, a result may be abnormal even if not flagged as abnormal by the laboratory or hospital electronic medical record. The magnitude of the abnormality should also be considered and can yield clues as to the etiology, although no direct correlation exists between aminotransferase levels and the degree of hepatic inflammation or fibrosis that are present. Mild to moderate elevations (30 to 150 U/L) are generally consistent with chronic liver disease, including NAFLD, chronic viral hepatitis, and other metabolic conditions such as alpha-1 antitrypsin deficiency, whereas more severe elevations can be suggestive of acute problems such as acute viral hepatitis, some medication toxicities, or hepatic ischemic injuries.

In addition to interpreting the initial laboratory values, one must also obtain information about the severity of possible liver disease. Clinical manifestations of liver disease can be subtle and require a more directed history and physical examination if not already performed. Questions should be targeted at detecting signs of liver dysfunction, such as a bleeding diathesis (bleeding when brushing teeth, frequent nosebleeds, easy bruising with minimal injury), a history of jaundice, and the presence of encephalopathy. It is important to recognize that encephalopathic change can be barely noticeable in its mildest form, involving reversal of sleep-wake cycles and mild cognitive deficits. Gastrointestinal bleeding is of particular significance, given that esophageal varices and hemorrhoids are specific complications that can result from cirrhosis and portal hypertension. Physical examination findings that suggest severe liver disease may be easy to miss and include hepatosplenomegaly, ascites, spider angioma, palmar erythema, and asterixis. If any evidence exists to suggest severe liver disease, an urgent referral should be made to a pediatric gastroenterologist.

Liver disease is oftentimes silent, without any overt symptoms or signs, and laboratory tests become essential indicators of what may otherwise be an indolent process. Part of characterizing the nature of that process involves assessing the trend of a test result over time because an abnormal ALT or AST elevation can be an acute and transient event or may be persistently elevated and thus signify a chronic pathology. Therefore, repeat measurement is recommended. With repeat measurement, resolution versus mild fluctuation versus worsening of aminotransferases over time becomes apparent, which both guides the differential diagnosis and influences the decision regarding referral to a specialist. Fractionated bilirubin (total and direct), alkaline phosphatase, and gamma-glutamyl transpeptidase are markers of hepatic cholestasis and biliary epithelial injury and will help to characterize the pattern of liver disease, and thus guide the differential diagnosis. Creatine kinase measurement will help determine whether the aminotransferase elevation is nonhepatic in origin. Ultimately, an important measure of whether a liver problem is an emergency is determined by the prothrombin time (PT)/international normalized ratio (INR) measurement. PT/INR is an objective parameter of hepatic synthetic function given that the liver is responsible for synthesis of clotting factors I, II, VII, and X, which PT measures. Liver failure is defined by an INR >2, or >1.5 if encephalopathy is present. Lastly, a complete blood count should also be checked, which can provide clues as to the presence of portal hypertension and splenomegaly because leukopenia and thrombocytopenia may be a result of splenic sequestration.

If aminotransferases are persistently elevated, referral to a specialist for further evaluation should be considered regardless of whether there are indicators of severe liver disease.[2] Although an elevated ALT in obese children often indicates fatty liver,[5] it is important to consider other conditions that might be causing the ALT elevation. NAFLD is indeed the most common cause of liver pathology in the obese population; however, elevated ALT does *not* equal an NAFLD diagnosis. A broad differential diagnosis must be considered, taking into account clinical context to guide further evaluation (Table 17-1). This is especially important when considering that some conditions are progressive and yet have directed and effective therapeutic interventions that can halt and even reverse the disease course (Table 17-2).

Table 17-1

Differential Diagnosis of Elevated Aminotransferase Activity in Obese Children and Adolescents

- Acute viral hepatitis
- Autoimmune hepatitis
- Alpha-1 antitrypsin deficiency
- Biliary obstruction *(choledocholithiasis)*
- Budd-Chiari syndrome
- Celiac disease
- Chronic viral hepatitis *(hepatitis B, hepatitis C, HIV)*
- Hemochromatosis
- Hepatic steatosis other than NAFLD
- Inflammatory bowel disease
- Ischemic injury
- Malignancies *(leukemia, lymphoma, liver tumors)*
- NAFLD
- Nonhepatic *(hemolysis, myopathy, strenuous exercise, macro-AST)*
- Toxic liver injury *(medications, supplements, alcohol, recreational drugs)*
- Thyroid disease
- Wilson's disease

Clinical history, including age, race/ethnicity, medications/supplements, and family history, is of particular importance to determine what other etiologies of hepatitis should be considered. For example, NAFLD is less common in children aged 9 years or younger.[1,6] Many medications can cause aminotransferase elevation, and a thorough history of medication use must be obtained. Moreover, it is extremely important to ask specifically about any over-the-counter, nutritional, naturopathic supplements, recreational drugs, or alcoholic substances that are being used that require immediate intervention with medication/supplement cessation and lifestyle modification. Viral hepatitis, autoimmune hepatitis, Wilson's disease, celiac disease, and alpha-1 antitrypsin deficiency are all conditions that may cause aminotransferase elevation in obese as well as non-obese individuals, and they should be screened for in the appropriate clinical context. Hepatitis A and B vaccination history and immune status should be determined followed by scheduled vaccination for those who are nonimmune. When evaluating elevated aminotransferases, a primary care provider must also recognize the importance of assessing for other comorbid conditions such as cardiovascular disease, endocrine abnormalities, or psychiatric conditions that may be present (see Questions 18, 22, and 27 for more details).

Although ultrasound is an attractive imaging modality because it is widely available, noninvasive without radiation exposure, and relatively inexpensive, its role in the evaluation and diagnosis of fatty liver is limited. Ultrasound has a poor sensitivity due to difficulty in detecting mild steatosis. The specificity is also not sufficiently robust because the positive predictive value is between

Table 17-2

Causes of Chronic Elevation in Aminotransferases Other Than NAFLD With Specific Interventions

Condition	Clinical Clue	Additional Screening Tests	Therapy
Alpha-1 antitrypsin deficiency	History of neonatal cholestasis, family history of early-onset emphysema	Alpha-1 antitrypsin phenotype	No specific therapy for liver; however, regular monitoring recommended; avoidance of smoking, second-hand smoke exposure to prevent pulmonary complications
Autoimmune hepatitis	Adolescent females, symptoms of fatigue, malaise	Antinuclear antibody, antismooth muscle antibody, anti-liver kidney microsomal antibody, quantitative immunoglobulin G	Steroids, immunomodulators
Celiac disease	Gastrointestinal complaints, associated condition (type 1 diabetes mellitus or thyroid disease), positive family history of celiac disease	Tissue transglutaminase IgA, quantitative IgA	Gluten-free diet
Chronic viral hepatitis	History of adoption, blood-product transfusion, tattoos, intravenous drug use, unprotected sexual intercourse	Hepatitis B surface antigen and antibody, hepatitis C antibody, HIV enzyme immunoassay	Targeted antiviral therapies
Wilson's disease	Neuropsychiatric symptoms, Kayser-Fleischer rings	Ceruloplasmin, 24-hour urinary copper	Trientine, penicillamine, zinc

47% and 62%. Definitive diagnosis for NAFLD and other conditions of the liver requires a liver biopsy. Of note, ultrasound has important strengths in detecting gallbladder and biliary pathology, an important comorbidity in the NAFLD population. In addition, ultrasound can be used to further evaluate complications of portal hypertension and presence of liver masses, which are of particular concern if cirrhosis is present.

Conclusion

Liver enzyme abnormalities in obese children and adolescents are common. ALT and AST measurement remains the best screening test available to identify children with liver disease, but does have certain limitations. An abnormal result may indicate a problem in the liver; however, it does not determine the nature of the problem, be it acute or chronic, the severity of the problem, or the etiology of the problem. A health care provider should be aware of these limitations and pursue further evaluation of the abnormality; consider referral to a specialist while watching for indications of an urgent issue. We have provided a suggested schematic representation of an approach to elevation in liver enzymes in the obese child to aid in navigation of this clinical situation (Figure 17-1).

References

1. Schwimmer JB, Deutsch R, Kahen T, Lavine JE, Stanley C, Behling C. Prevalence of fatty liver in children and adolescents. *Pediatrics*. 2006;118(4):1388-1393.
2. Barlow SE; Expert Committee. Expert committee recommendations regarding the prevention, assessment, and treatment of child and adolescent overweight and obesity: summary report. *Pediatrics*. 2007;120(Suppl 4): S164-S192.
3. Schwimmer JB. Definitive diagnosis and assessment of risk for nonalcoholic fatty liver disease in children and adolescents. *Semin Liver Dis*. 2007;27(3):312-318.
4. Schwimmer JB, Dunn W, Norman GJ, et al. SAFETY study: alanine aminotransferase cutoff values are set too high for reliable detection of pediatric chronic liver disease. *Gastroenterology*. 2010;138(4):1357-1364, 1364.e1-1364.e2.
5. Fishbein MH, Miner M, Mogren C, Chalekson J. The spectrum of fatty liver in obese children and the relationship of serum aminotransferases to severity of steatosis. *J Pediatr Gastroenterol Nutr*. 2003;36(1): 54-61.
6. Schwimmer JB, McGreal N, Deutsch R, Finegold MJ, Lavine JE. Influence of gender, race, and ethnicity on suspected fatty liver in obese adolescents. *Pediatrics*. 2005;115(5): e561-e565.

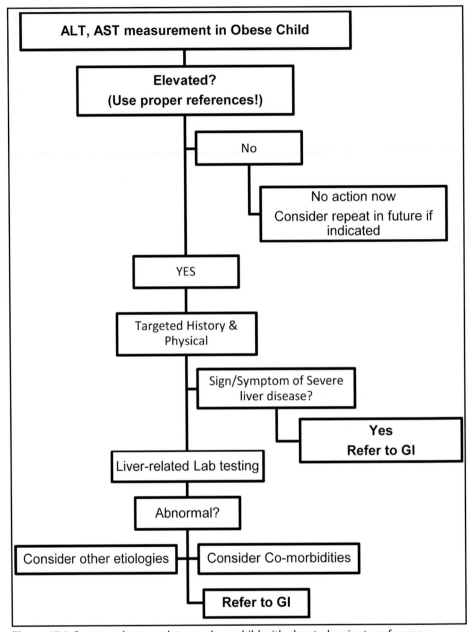

Figure 17-1. Suggested approach to an obese child with elevated aminotransferases.

18
QUESTION

WHAT IS THE RELATIONSHIP BETWEEN DIABETES AND PEDIATRIC OBESITY?

Andrei Fodoreanu, MD and Michael Gottschalk, MD, PhD

The relationship between diabetes and pediatric obesity is a complex one, including gene and early life environment interactions, timing of weight gain, body composition, familial risk factors, and economic factors. As we will see next, subclinical chronic systemic inflammation may be the most important factor defining this relationship and the missing link between diabetes and pediatric obesity.

Obesity is strongly related to type 2 diabetes (T2D) in pediatric patients as opposed to type 1 diabetes (T1D). Children affected by T2D are found to be obese when compared with nonaffected children, and this is in contrast with children affected by T1D, who have a higher prevalence of being overweight but are not obese. It is also important to note that T2D has been found to be associated with a strong family history of diabetes, has a higher prevalence in girls and ethnic minorities, and is mostly present in a household with an annual income less than $25,000, with a highest parent/guardian education level of less than a high school degree, and in the context of lacking a family structure.

T2D is the result of the combined states of insulin resistance (IR) and a beta cell insulin secretory defect. Obesity is one of the most important causes in development of IR, and subsequently T2D. IR is the inability of physiologic levels of insulin to transport glucose into the cells, suppress gluconeogenesis in the liver, and lipolysis in the fat cells. As such, IR is the best predictor of impaired glucose tolerance (IGT), a pre-T2D condition. Individuals with IGT have a 10% rate per year of developing T2D. Lipotoxicity and body weight gain have an important role in the development of IR. Interestingly, it is the accumulation of muscle fat (intramyocellular fat) and visceral fat, as opposed to peripheral subcutaneous fat accumulation, that seems to cause IR and subsequently IGT and T2D. The deposition of fat in other organs, such as into the liver or pancreas, also has a significant detrimental effect, leading, for example, to secretory defects of the pancreatic B-cells, causing a decrease in insulin production. The exact molecular mechanism has not been completely

Huang JS, ed. *Curbside Consultation in
Pediatric Obesity: 49 Clinical Questions* (pp 83-84).
© 2014 Taylor & Francis Group

elucidated but seems to involve an increase in oxidative stress in target tissues, affecting the endoplasmic reticulum and mitochondrial function of affected cells.

Metabolic imprinting by the perinatal environment may play a role in the development of diabetes for some individuals. Epidemiologic data demonstrate that, in the case of small-for-gestational-age babies, there is an increased risk of developing both diabetes and obesity due to prenatal developmental adaptive responses that ensure survival and growth in a nutrient-poor environment (ie, malnourished mothers). Such adaptive responses then persist after birth but become detrimental in a nutrient-rich environment, leading to parallel development of diabetes and obesity.

The multiple factors leading to IR continue to be described, but among all underlying molecular processes involved, subclinical chronic systemic inflammation in the setting of obesity is the most independently associated. Muscle and visceral adipocytes, in response to excess lipid storage, secrete increasing amounts of inflammatory cytokines and chemokines, leading to migration of macrophages to these adipose tissues, which in turn leads to further increase in cytokine release, initiating a proinflammatory state. This is an important point to remember: the presence of obesity leads to production of proinflammatory cytokines. Furthermore, in response to the increased amount of stored lipids, the adipocytes secrete less anti-inflammatory peptides such as adiponectin, which has the opposite effect and confers insulin sensitivity. As such, the balance is tipped toward systemic inflammation, and this can be demonstrated by high levels of inflammatory markers such as C-reactive protein, which, driven by increasing cytokine interleukin-6 concentrations, have been found in obese children and strongly correlate and predict T2D. Therefore, systemic inflammation appears to be the important link between pediatric obesity and T2D.

Before the 1990s, T2D was a rare pediatric disease, but by 1999, new cases of T2D in children and adolescents ranged from 8% to 45% depending on geographic area. Recent population-based data indicate that T2D is diagnosed in approximately 1 in 3700 children and adolescents annually, and at the current rising rates in obesity, the Centers for Disease Control predicts that 1 in 3 babies will develop diabetes in their lifetime (with an even higher incidence in African American and Hispanic children). Data collected also found that T2D has been presenting with an increasing prevalence in children, in parallel with the high prevalence of pediatric obesity. The early presentation of T2D in the pediatric population suggests an accelerated process of disease development, with a shorter transition time between IGT and T2D as compared with adults. T2D in children seems to be a more aggressive disease than in adults and encompasses a rapid failure of pancreatic B-cell function, with studies even demonstrating a higher rate of metformin treatment failure in children than in adults. Obesity leading to IR may unmask a prediabetic phenotype present in the affected pediatric population. This rapid transition in children from normal glucose tolerance to IGT and then to T2D is highly associated with significant increases in weight and relative adiposity, independent of ethnicity, sex, and pubertal status, suggesting that obesity prevention is an important area of preventive intervention for diabetes as well. Given the notably increased risk for T2D with early weight gain, early intervention and obesity prevention are key roles for the pediatrician to play in T2D prevention.

Suggested Readings

D'Adamo E, Caprio S. Type 2 diabetes in youth: epidemiology and pathophysiology. *Diabetes Care.* 2011;34(Suppl 2):S161-S165.

DeBoer MD. Obesity, systemic inflammation, and increased risk for cardiovascular disease and diabetes among adolescents: a need for screening tools to target interventions. *Nutrition.* 2013;29(2):379-386.

Han JC, Lawlor DA, Kimm SY. Childhood obesity. *Lancet.* 2010;375(9727):1737-1748.

Weiss R, Caprio S. The metabolic consequences of childhood obesity. *Best Pract Res Clin Endocrinol Metab.* 2005;19(3): 405-419.

Weiss R, Dziura J, Burgert TS, et al. Obesity and the metabolic syndrome in children and adolescents. *N Engl J Med.* 2004;350(23):2362-2374.

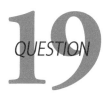

WHAT ARE THE COMMON ORTHOPEDIC ISSUES IN THE OBESE CHILD?

Heather M. Kong, MD and Sanjeev Sabharwal, MD, MPH

Childhood obesity is an increasingly common problem with health implications affecting several organ systems, including the musculoskeletal system. Primary care physicians and specialists should be aware of the various orthopedic issues that are more prevalent among obese youth. Because of these children's excessive body mass index (BMI), large amounts of mechanical loads are constantly placed on the weight-bearing joints of the lower extremities, often leading to premature arthritis of the hips and knees. Compared with their leaner peers, obese children are more likely to complain of back, knee, and foot pain. Given their large thigh girth and increased prevalence of painful flat feet, these children walk with an abnormal gait, often dragging their feet, which are pointed outward.[1,2]

Certain pediatric orthopedic disorders, such as slipped capital femoral epiphysis (SCFE) and Blount disease, are more often seen in obese children and adolescents. Although the exact etiology of these developmental disorders is likely multifactorial, a sustained increase in the mechanical load at certain growth plates of the lower extremity is probably the major contributing factor. Owing to their central obesity, these children are also predisposed to sustaining distal extremity fractures.

Slipped Capital Femoral Epiphysis

SCFE is the posteromedial displacement of the proximal femoral epiphysis relative to the femoral neck and shaft. Mean age at presentation is 13.5 years for boys and 12 years for girls. The majority of affected children are aged 10 to 16 years at the time of clinical presentation. While other predispositions such as ethnicity (eg, African American, Polynesian populations) and

Huang JS, ed. *Curbside Consultation in Pediatric Obesity: 49 Clinical Questions* (pp 85-89).
© 2014 Taylor & Francis Group

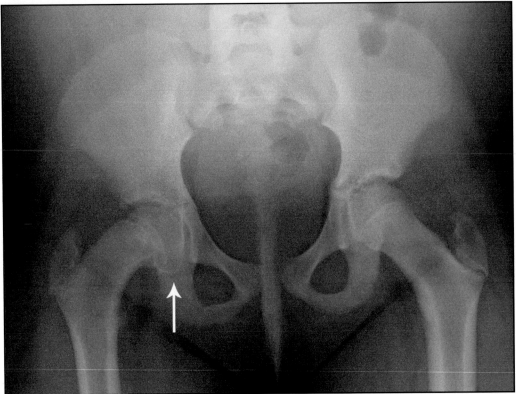

Figure 19-1. Anteroposterior radiograph of the pelvis of a 12-year-old obese girl demonstrating an SCFE (arrow) of the right side. She had a 3-month history of insidious onset of right knee and thigh discomfort. Physical examination demonstrated an out-toeing gait on the right with decreased internal rotation and excessive external rotation of the right compared with the left hip.

endocrine abnormalities (eg, hypothyroidism, hypopituitarism) may contribute, obesity is assumed to be the main risk factor for developing SCFE. Studies have shown that up to 70% of children are above the 80th percentile for weight, and about 50% of those diagnosed are above the 90th percentile.[3] Based on reports from several countries, the prevalence of SCFE, including bilateral disease, is increasing. The growing number of cases is speculated to be closely related to the rising rates of childhood obesity in these regions.[1]

Patients with SCFE typically present with an insidious onset of hip or knee (referred) pain along with a progressively worsening limp. Physical examination findings typically include a limp and limited mobility of the affected hip(s), especially internal rotation. Obligate external rotation with flexion of the involved hip is a hallmark of SCFE. Given the possibility of an asymptomatic contralateral slip, the examiner should be vigilant and perform clinical and radiographic evaluation of both hips. Radiographic studies should include an anteroposterior view of the pelvis and lateral views of both hips (Figures 19-1 and 19-2). Although SCFEs were historically classified as acute or chronic based on the duration of symptoms (greater or less than 3 weeks), classification as stable or unstable provides a better prognostic indicator. A child who can still bear weight on the affected limb (even with a limp or with an assistive device) is considered to have a stable slip, as opposed to a patient who cannot bear any weight (unstable). Unstable SCFEs have been associated with a significantly higher rate of avascular necrosis of the femoral head (up to 50% [unstable] versus approximately 1% [stable]).[3]

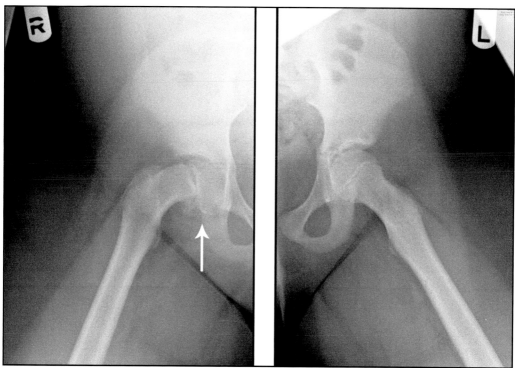

Figure 19-2. Lateral view radiographs of the same child in Figure 19-1 demonstrating the SCFE (arrow) of the right hip and normal appearance of the left hip. Given the possibility of bilaterality, both hips were visualized to rule out an asymptomatic contralateral SCFE. She underwent an urgent in situ pinning of the right SCFE.

Based on natural history studies, patients with SCFE are predisposed to premature arthritis of the affected hip joint. Since the severity and duration of symptoms are directly related to the amount of "slip" of the femoral epiphysis, it is crucial to prevent further progression of the SCFE. To minimize this risk of progression, the child suspected of having SCFE should be urgently referred to an orthopedic surgeon for definitive management. Referral to the emergency room is actually more appropriate than an office setting because this problem requires prompt surgical treatment. The patient should also be placed on crutches or provided a wheelchair, with no weightbearing on the affected limb(s). Surgery typically involves percutaneous in situ screw fixation into the femoral head and neck to prevent further displacement of the epiphysis. In cases of bilateral SCFE, both sides are surgically treated in the same operative session. Although somewhat controversial, certain authors also recommend prophylactic surgical fixation of the contralateral, uninvolved hip in patients with unilateral SCFE.

Blount Disease

Blount disease[4] (also known as *tibia vara*) is a developmental disorder primarily affecting the medial portion of the upper end of the growing tibia. Blount disease is classified based on the age of onset of the lower leg deformity, as early onset (< 4 years old) and late onset (> 4 years old). Patients with early-onset Blount disease are more likely to have bilateral involvement and more severe deformities than late-onset patients (Figures 19-3 and 19-4). A strong correlation has been

Figure 19-3. Clinical photo of an 8-year-old obese girl with bilateral genu varum secondary to early-onset Blount disease. She had progressive bowing of both knees starting at age 2 years.

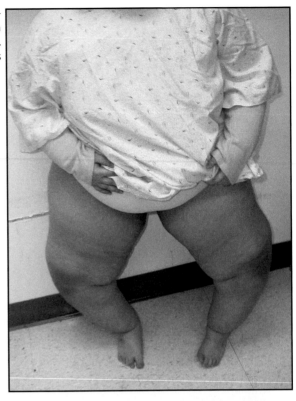

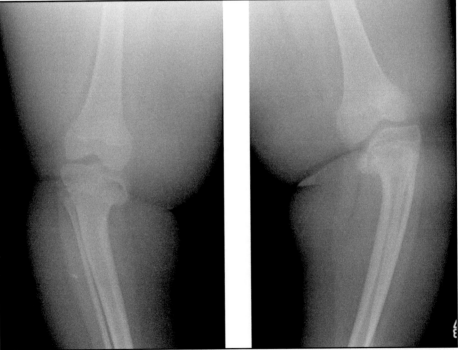

Figure 19-4. Anteroposterior radiograph of both knees of the obese child with Blount disease shown in Figure 19-3. Besides the genu varum, irregularity of the medial aspect of the proximal tibial growth plate (physis) is also noted.

established between the child's BMI and Blount disease. Although the pathogenesis is multifactorial, excessive mechanical loading is thought to play an important role in this asymmetric physeal growth. The increase in mechanical loads noted in the posteromedial aspect of the proximal tibial physis leads to a progressive 3-dimensional deformity involving varus, procurvatum, and internal rotation of the affected lower leg. Thus, the child presents with bowlegs and in-toeing. These clinical findings are consistent with a well-known biologic phenomenon of growth inhibition related to excessive compressive forces across the growth plate, known as the *Hueter-Volkmann principle*. Blount disease is often associated with gait abnormalities and leg-length discrepancy, and, if left untreated, may eventually lead to premature arthritis of the knee.

Blount disease patients are usually brought in by their caretakers with concerns for bowlegs, with or without knee pain. This clinical entity must be distinguished from physiologic bowing, especially in young children, which typically resolves by 2 years of age. Physical examination demonstrates genu varum and internal tibial torsion, often with shortening of the involved extremity. Radiographic examination almost always confirms the diagnosis. A full-length standing anteroposterior radiograph of both lower extremities is obtained to assess the mechanical axis of each lower limb, as well as radiographs of the affected tibia. Typical radiographic findings include widening and irregularity of the medial proximal tibial physis; some of the bowing deformity may be related to varus deformity of the distal femur. Computed tomography scan and magnetic resonance imaging may also be used to further assess the extent of disease and for preoperative planning. Treatment of Blount disease depends on the age of the patient, severity of deformity, and leg-length discrepancy. Although nonoperative treatment can be attempted with orthoses, the natural history of the disease is one of progressively worsening deformity. Surgical options include guided growth (hemiepiphysiodesis of the lateral aspect of the proximal tibia and/or distal femur) and valgus osteotomy of the proximal tibia with either acute or gradual correction (using distraction osteogenesis). A variety of implants, such as plates and screws or external fixation, can be used to maintain the correction. Obese children are less likely to obtain adequate correction from less invasive guided-growth procedures and may require more extensive surgical correction.

Perioperative Considerations

In addition to a predisposition for certain orthopedic problems and injuries, obese children are also at higher risk for some perioperative complications. These individuals generally require a longer operative time and have longer inpatient hospital stays than their peers. Obese patients are more prone to obstructive sleep apnea, difficult intubation, and intraoperative oxygen desaturation, which the accompanying anesthesiologist must be aware of. Despite the extra soft tissue padding, overweight and obese children are also more prone to developing pressure ulcers, both intraoperatively and postoperatively. Wound complications and infections are more prevalent as well. Because obesity is also a risk factor for venous thromboembolism, consideration should be given to mechanical and/or chemical thromboembolic prophylaxis, even in pediatric patients.

References

1. Gettys FK, Jackson JB, Frick SL. Obesity in pediatric orthopaedics. *Orthop Clin North Am.* 2011;42(1):95-105.
2. Sabharwal S, Root MZ. Impact of obesity on orthopaedics. *J Bone Joint Surg Am.* 2012;94(11):1045-1052.
3. Morrissy RT, Weinstein S, eds. *Lovell and Winter's Pediatric Orthopaedics.* Philadelphia, PA: Lippincott Williams & Wilkins; 2006.
4. Sabharwal S. Blount disease. *J Bone Joint Surg Am.* 2009;91(7):1758-1776.

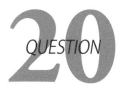

DOES OBESITY AFFECT REPRODUCTION? HOW?

Kimberly Henrichs, MD and Ellen L. Connor, MD

Obesity affects all stages of reproduction and negatively affects fertility in both women and men (Table 20-1). Effects of obesity on sexual development and reproduction begin as early as infancy. Rapid weight gain in early life is associated with precocious puberty. Increased body mass index (BMI) in adolescence is clearly associated with earlier pubertal development in females. The effects of elevated BMI on male pubertal onset are less clear. Some studies suggest that male obesity is related to earlier voice break and puberty, whereas others highlight a subgroup of boys in whom obesity appears to attenuate puberty.[1]

During the reproductive years, obesity in women is associated with increased risk of anovulatory cycles, decreased conceptions per ovulatory cycle, and increased time to spontaneous conception in ovulating females.[2,3] The pathophysiology is thought to be related to hyperinsulinemia and elevated adipokines, hormones secreted by adipose cells. Insulin resistance (IR) and hyperinsulinemia increase as visceral fat mass increases. High insulin levels inhibit liver production of sex hormone-binding globulin (SHBG). SHBG is important to bind androgens and decrease their apparent effect on women. High insulin also stimulates testosterone and dehydroepiandrostenedione production by ovarian theca cells, resulting in increased free androgens. These androgens may be peripherally converted to estrogen, increasing negative feedback inhibition of the hypothalamic-pituitary-ovary axis that leads to oligoovulation/anovulation. Combined effects of hyperinsulinemia and hyperandrogenemia may further inhibit fertility by promoting granulosa cell death and premature follicular atresia.

In men, obesity may secondarily worsen preexisting fertility issues, rather than play a primary role in male infertility. However, obesity rates are higher among males with poor semen quality.[4] Several studies have evaluated the relationship between obesity and sperm parameters with conflicting results. The link between male obesity and endocrine dysfunction is more defined.

Huang JS, ed. *Curbside Consultation in Pediatric Obesity: 49 Clinical Questions* (pp 91-94). © 2014 Taylor & Francis Group

Table 20-1
Effects of Obesity on Reproduction Across the Lifetime

Childhood

Advanced puberty
- Delayed puberty in a subset of males

Reproductive Years
- Increased anovulatory cycles
- Decreased conception per ovulation
- Increased time to conception
- ± Altered sperm integrity
- Altered testosterone-to-estrogen ratio

Maternal Effects During Pregnancy

Increased risk of:
- Early miscarriage
- Fetal demise
- Recurrent miscarriages
- Hypertension
- Preeclampsia
- Gestational diabetes
- Venous thrombosis
- Genital/urinary tract infections
- Induction of labor
- Failure to progress
- Instrumental delivery
- Transition to emergent cesarean section
- Failed trial of labor after prior cesarean section
- Wound infection
- Difficulties with lactation

Fetal Effects During Pregnancy

Increases risk of:
- Large-for-gestational-age infant
  - Abnormal presentation
  - Dystocia
  - Injury during delivery
  - Neonatal hypoglycemia
- Congenital anomalies
  - Cardiovascular
  - Renal
  - Neural tube
- Elective premature delivery

Infancy

Increased lifetime risk of obesity

Similar to females, obese males have lower SHBG levels related to hyperinsulinemia. The paucity of SHBG results in lower total testosterone and free testosterone. Peripheral conversion of unbound testosterone to estradiol can shift the testosterone:estradiol ratio. A decreased testosterone:estradiol ratio is associated with infertility. Although only a subgroup of obese males have hypogonadotropic hypogonadism (central inability to produce gonadotropins), mild increases in estradiol may interrupt the hypothalamic-pituitary-testis axis by dampening luteinizing hormone pulses and bioactivity.

Leptin is the best understood adipokine affecting reproduction. Leptin levels are elevated in obesity. In females, leptin inhibits ovarian follicle development and granulosa cell estradiol production. Leptin may also counteract insulin-induced steroid hormone synthesis in theca and granulosa cells.[2] In males, leptin receptors are located on the testicular Leydig cells and spermatozoa. Leptin levels may affect sperm function and quality.[4]

Any discussion on the effects of obesity in reproductive years should include polycystic ovary syndrome (PCOS). PCOS is the most common endocrine disorder of reproductive age, occurring in 5% to 12% of females.[5] PCOS is defined clinically by irregular or absent ovulation, androgen excess demonstrated in blood or on examination, and/or radiographic findings of polycystic ovaries, after excluding other causes. Clinical hyperandrogenism can be identified by hirsutism (excess terminal hair growth in androgen-dependent areas such as the face, chest, and abdomen), acne, or male-pattern baldness. Patients with PCOS are at increased risk for metabolic syndrome. The incidence of obesity in adult women with PCOS is as high as 60%.[3] Obese females with PCOS are more likely to have anovulation and poor response to pharmacological induction of ovulation.

Even after conception occurs, obesity adds risks and complications. Obese women have higher rates of early miscarriage, fetal demise after 28 weeks' gestation, and recurrent miscarriages. Obesity in pregnancy is associated with increased incidence of hypertension, preeclampsia, gestational diabetes, venous thrombosis, and genital/urinary tract infections. Although spontaneous premature birth is less common in infants of obese women, these women still have an increased risk for elective premature delivery secondary to other factors. At the time of expected delivery, obese women have higher incidences of requiring induction of labor, as well as failure to progress, instrumental delivery, and transition to emergent cesarean section. Obesity is also a risk factor for failed trial of labor after prior cesarean section. In the perinatal period, obesity confers a greater chance of wound infection and lactation difficulties.[2,3]

Mothers are not the only ones affected by obesity in pregnancy. An intrauterine environment that is altered by hyperglycemia, hyperinsulinemia with IR, and hyperandrogenemia may have epigenetic effects on offspring. These offspring have an increased lifetime risk of obesity. Intrauterine hyperglycemia results in an increased frequency of large-for-gestational-age infants and subsequent increased risk for abnormal presentation, dystocia, injury during delivery, and neonatal hypoglycemia. Obesity also confers increased risk of congenital anomalies, including cardiovascular, renal, and neural tube defects, which are less often detected prenatally than in average-weight pregnancies. Interestingly, prenatal folic acid supplementation has less-protective benefits in preventing congenital anomalies in obese pregnancies compared with normal weight pregnancies.[2]

Given the increasing magnitude of obesity and its transgenerational impacts, health care professionals must prevent and treat obesity. First and foremost, patients should be empowered with education. Obese patients should be counseled on the benefits of weight loss before conception. Even as little as a 5% to 10% weight loss can improve long-term health outcomes. The cornerstone to sustained weight loss and weight management is lifestyle changes, including diet and exercise. At present, a low-carbohydrate diet appears more effective for weight loss than one focused on low-fat intake for IR patients.[2] Studies of women with PCOS demonstrate improved menstrual cyclicity, ovulatory frequency, and pregnancy outcomes with successful weight loss. The ideal timing of weight loss for reproduction is not defined, although some studies suggest that periconceptual dieting may lead to increased risk of pre-term births. For this reason, and to counter the adverse effects of obesity on offspring, patients should achieve weight loss before conception. The addition of pharmacological weight-loss agents is helpful for acute weight loss but is questionable in women actively trying to conceive. No evidence supports enduring benefits of these medications in many patients.

Assisted reproduction is available for obese women unable to conceive independently. Clomiphene citrate, an anti-estrogen that raises serum follicle-stimulating hormone levels to stimulate follicular growth and development, is presently first-line pharmacological therapy. Clomiphene results in conception rates up to 50% following 3 to 6 cycles of therapy; conception rates increase to 75% after 9 cycles.[3] The addition of metformin to clomiphene may not increase pregnancy rates in obese PCOS women, although some studies have shown increased rates of spontaneous conception and live births in PCOS-affected women taking metformin.[6] Gonadotropins (namely follicle-stimulating hormone) are preferred second-line therapy for assisted reproduction. However, obese women frequently require longer periods of stimulation and greater total doses of gonadotropins to conceive, which places them at increased risk for multiple gestations and ovarian hyperstimulation syndrome. If clomiphene and gonadotropins fail, in vitro fertilization remains an option. Obese women who undergo in vitro fertilization do not show increased miscarriages compared with normal weight women.

Evidence-based pharmacological options for obese subfertile males are limited. Aromatase inhibitors, which prevent the peripheral conversion of testosterone to estradiol, may normalize testosterone levels and decrease estradiol.[4] However, available studies are limited by small sample sizes and lack appropriate controls to discern applicable effects. The effects of anti-estrogens ± testosterone undecanoate may improve spermatogenesis and fertility in some normal-weight males with idiopathic oligospermia, but no studies have specifically examined outcomes in obese males.[4]

Obesity affects all phases of human reproduction. Initially obesity appears to accelerate maturation in females and many males, followed by an attenuation of reproductive capacity. Although many obese individuals conceive and reproduce without complication, obesity imparts increased risk for many adverse health outcomes and severely challenges reproductive attempts. Given the significance of these effects, we recommend focused efforts on obesity prevention and treatment before conception.

References

1. Wagner IV, Sabin MA, Pfäffle RW, et al. Effects of obesity on human sexual development. *Nat Rev Endocrinol.* 2012;8(4):246-254.
2. Metwally M, Li TC, Ledger WL. The impact of obesity on female reproductive function. *Obes Rev.* 2007;8(6):515-523.
3. Nelson SM, Fleming R. Obesity and reproduction: impact and interventions. *Curr Opin Obstet Gynecol.* 2007;19(4):384-389.
4. Teerds KJ, de Rooij DG, Keijer J. Functional relationship between obesity and male reproduction: from humans to animal models. *Hum Reprod Update.* 2011;17(5):667-683.
5. March WA, Moore VM, Willson KJ, Phillips DI, Norman RJ, Davies MJ. The prevalence of polycystic ovary syndrome in a community sample assessed under contrasting diagnostic criteria. *Hum Reprod.* 2010;25(2):544-551.
6. Glueck CJ, Goldenberg N, Pranikoff J, Khan Z, Padda J, Wang P. Effects of metformin-diet intervention before and throughout pregnancy on obstetric and neonatal outcomes in patients with polycystic ovary syndrome. *Curr Med Res Opin.* 2013;29(1):55-62.

21
QUESTION

MANY OF MY PEDIATRIC PATIENTS COMPLAIN ABOUT FATIGUE. WHAT CONDITIONS SHOULD I BE ESPECIALLY CONCERNED ABOUT IN MY OBESE PATIENTS?

Christopher Davis, MD, PhD

Obese children commonly complain of being fatigued, tired, and/or sleepy throughout the course of the day. In addition, they often complain of excessive fatigue during exercise and have a general lack of tolerance for exercise and decreased endurance compared with their peers. Several factors can contribute to these symptoms, all of which should be considered and addressed if present. Although the ultimate treatment for these symptoms is to fix the underlying problem of obesity itself and contributors to its development, simply changing behavior can begin to have an impact on levels of fatigue, independent of weight loss.

Chronic daytime fatigue and sleepiness can affect obese children through several mechanisms. Obstructive sleep apnea (OSA) is often thought of as a primary cause for daytime sleepiness. OSA is present in approximately 3% of children aged 2 to 8 years.[1] Indeed, OSA should be ruled out in the initial evaluation of daytime sleepiness because treatment (in addition to weight loss) is available in the form of positive airway pressure.[2] However, it must be recognized that sleepiness and fatigue are also prevalent among obese patients without sleep apnea, and in fact these symptoms are usually not caused by OSA.[3] Obese persons generally have poorer sleep quality than normal-weight individuals. They may also have one or more comorbid conditions that require consideration. First, insulin resistance (and diabetes) is a known cause of fatigue and is prevalent in obese patients. Measurement of fasting glucose and/or more involved measures of insulin sensitivity should be undertaken if this is suspected. Second, women with polycystic ovarian syndrome (itself associated with insulin resistance) will often complain of daytime sleepiness. This condition, although heterogeneous, is characterized by hyperandrogenism and chronic anovulation. Third, lack of physical activity is associated with daytime fatigue and sleepiness. Physical activity levels can be measured to some degree, but a simple history can allow a good approximation of exercise

Huang JS, ed. *Curbside Consultation in Pediatric Obesity: 49 Clinical Questions* (pp 95-96).

frequency, amount of sitting time, and overall level of activity. Increasing one's level of daily physical activity can help reduce symptoms of fatigue, and this occurs independently of weight, presence of sleep apnea, and metabolic status. Finally, and importantly, a significant association exists between fatigue/sleepiness and depression among obese patients. Thus, screening for mood disorders is essential when confronted with an obese patient complaining of excessive daytime sleepiness and fatigue.

A different but related symptom common in obese children is excessive fatigue during exercise or simply poor exercise tolerance. This symptom also has several potential causes.[4] The first is that there is a higher energy requirement for movement when an individual has excessive adipose tissue. During weightbearing exercise, muscles must perform extra work to move a greater total body mass. This causes earlier fatigue than in normal-weight individuals. There is also an increased metabolic cost of breathing when the respiratory muscles are required to move the excessive mass of the chest wall in obese patients. The fatigue and associated discomfort that arises during exercise for these patients often results in reduced physical activity levels because patients learn to avoid the unpleasant feelings associated with exercise. This causes a pathologic cycle of decreasing levels of physical activity, often accompanied by more weight gain and decreased exercise tolerance and even further discomfort with attempted exercise. Breaking the cycle requires consistent physical activity and eventual weight loss. It is important to stress to obese patients that they should exercise as much as possible, independent of weight loss, because the salutary benefits of exercise occur in individuals throughout a large range of body mass. These include improved insulin sensitivity, improved confidence and mood, and healthier skeletal muscle, to name a few.

Although uncommon, other causes of exercise-related symptoms in obese patients that often accompany fatigue, such as dyspnea, dizziness, and chest discomfort, should be considered. Obesity itself does not preclude underlying pulmonary and/or cardiac pathology. Exercise-induced asthma is not uncommon, and in fact obesity and asthma are often comorbid conditions. Even obese nonasthmatics can have bronchospasm induced by exercise, which may further limit overall physical activity by causing discomfort during exercise. Various forms of heart disease can present as exertional dyspnea and fatigue. Examples include cardiomyopathies, congenital coronary anomalies (which more often cause exertional chest pain or syncope), myocarditis, and other structural heart disease such as valvular disease. Fortunately, these conditions are relatively rare. The most likely reason by far for exertional dyspnea and discomfort is obesity itself and the commonly associated deconditioned state of those individuals. Obtaining a family history to uncover the presence of cardiac and pulmonary disease in young relatives and performing a proper physical examination are adequate for purposes of screening for heart and lung disease. Further tests should be performed only if indicated. For instance, a bronchodilator challenge may be prudent for patients with wheezing or cough during exercise. Referral to a pulmonary or cardiovascular specialist may be indicated if these specific signs or symptoms exist.

References

1. Tauman R, Gozal D. Obstructive sleep apnea in children. *Paediatr Resp Rev.* 2006;7(4):247-259.
2. Vgontzas AN, Kales A. Sleep and its disorders. *Annu Rev Med.* 1999;50:387-400.
3. Vgontzas AN, Bixler EO, Chrousos GP. Obesity-related sleepiness and fatigue: the role of the stress system and cytokines. *Ann N Y Acad Sci.* 2006;1083:329-344.
4. Whipp BJ, Davis JA. The ventilatory stress of exercise in obesity. *Am Rev Respir Dis.* 1984;129(2 Pt 2):S90-S92.

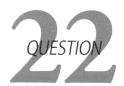

OBESITY IS ASSOCIATED WITH CARDIOVASCULAR DISEASE IN ADULTS. IS THIS TRUE IN CHILDREN? HOW WOULD I DIAGNOSE CARDIOVASCULAR COMPLICATIONS IN THE OBESE CHILD?

Paul W. Franks, BSc(Hons), MS, MPhil (Cantab), PhD (Cantab), FTOS
and Angela Estampador, BS, MPH

Obesity is a major risk factor for metabolic and cardiovascular disease in adults. The Framingham Heart Study was established to follow the development of cardiovascular disease (CVD) over a long period of time and to identify major risk factors for premature death.[1] The study was one of the first to show that obesity is a major risk factor for CVD in adults.

Epidemiological data have shown in recent years that, as in adulthood, childhood obesity also raises the risk of metabolic disease and CVD later in life and consequently shortens lifespan.[2] The Bogalusa Heart Study is a long-term prospective cohort study in children that has provided some of the most robust epidemiological evidence that the etiology of adult heart disease often stems from childhood.[3] In another longitudinal study of 230,000 Norwegian adolescents, Bjørge et al found that individuals in the highest 2 body mass index (BMI) categories (85th to 94th and ≥ 95th percentiles based on Centers for Disease Control growth charts in the United States) had a higher risk of death from metabolic and circulatory diseases, and those in the highest BMI category had an increased risk of death from ischemic heart disease as compared with their normal-weight (25th to 75th percentile BMI) counterparts.[4]

CVD is caused to a large extent by the accumulation of lipids within the blood that cause atherosclerotic plaques to form, thickening the arterial walls with consequential narrowing of the arteries. Hypertension, defined as chronically elevated blood pressure (BP), may promote this process and itself be a primary risk factor for CVD, particularly myocardial infarction, abdominal aortic aneurysm, and hemorrhagic stroke, or secondary to other risk factors including atherosclerosis. Hypertension is defined by BP (either systolic or diastolic) percentiles using the following cutoff points in children and adolescents:

- *Prehypertensive* when equal to the 90th but less than 95th percentiles or if BP exceeds 120/80 mm Hg

Huang JS, ed. *Curbside Consultation in Pediatric Obesity: 49 Clinical Questions* (pp 97-101).
© 2014 Taylor & Francis Group

- *Stage 1 hypertensive* when between the 90th and 99th percentiles plus 5 mm Hg

- *Stage 2 hypertensive* when greater than the 99th percentile plus 5 mm Hg

Please refer to the US Department of Health & Human Services National Heart, Lung and Blood Institute (NHLBI) Blood Pressure Tables with percentiles by age, sex, and height in the *Fourth Report on the Diagnosis, Evaluation, and Treatment of High Blood Pressure in Children and Adolescents.*[5] Atherosclerosis is highly prevalent in older adults but also occurs sometimes in childhood, particularly in obese children, making this population subgroup an important focus for primary prevention.[6] The Pathobiological Determinants of Atherosclerosis in Youth Study (PDAY) began in 1985 to study risk factors for coronary heart disease in young people.[7] The study contributed greatly to our current understanding of atherosclerotic disease and notably documented the disease's natural progression in adolescents and young adults, using autopsied aortic and coronary artery specimens obtained from medical centers throughout the United States.[6] The PDAY study provided some of the first concrete evidence that atherosclerosis can occur before adulthood.

The rate of atherosclerosis progression in children and young adults, as marked by the presence, number, and severity of fatty streaks and fibrous plaques in the aorta and coronary arteries, corresponds with the number of CVD risk factors present in the child, with an increasing number of risk factors conferring a cumulative effect on the risk of disease.[8] These CVD risk factors include high age-sex standardized BMI, elevated systolic BP, elevated triacylglycerol inflammatory cytokines, and elevated low-density lipoprotein (LDL) cholesterol levels in the blood (values above the 75th percentile are considered high/elevated).[8] An additional risk factor is a positive family history of CVD.

Dyslipidemia (elevated triglycerides and LDL-cholesterol and low high-density lipoprotein (HDL)-cholesterol concentrations; Table 22-1) in childhood can trigger the development of atherosclerosis in genetically susceptible children requiring that they adhere to careful dietary practices aimed at reducing the intake of saturated fats. Whether dyslipidemia in children who are obese and who do not carry hyperlipidogenic mutations causes subsequent heart disease is less clear. For example, childhood BMI and hypertension were strongly associated with premature cardiovascular mortality (before age 55 years) in a prospective cohort study of overweight and obese children, but hypercholesterolemia was not.[2] One limitation of this study is that lipid data were limited to total cholesterol, which may mask the effects of lipid subclasses and tells us little about the effects of triacylglycerols.

In late 2012, the NHLBI's Expert Panel on Integrated Guidelines for Cardiovascular and Risk Reduction in Children and Adolescents advocated for universal lipid screening between the ages of 9 and 11 years.[9] The task force recommends that lipid assessment (see Table 22-1) in children should ideally occur prior to puberty, when lipid and lipoprotein concentrations are most stable. Changes in lipid and lipoprotein levels are normally seen during puberty and can convolute the interpretation of future CVD risk; and tracking of lipid and lipoprotein levels in pediatric cohort studies shows that a significant decline in levels occurs after age 10 years (around the time of puberty in the US population) as part of the process of normal growth and development.[9] The guidelines state that lipid screening before age 9 years is warranted only if the child is obese (BMI ≥95th percentile of age-sex standardized distribution) and the child is characterized by one or more of the following additional factors: a family history of CVD, at least one dyslipidemic parent (total cholesterol ≥240 mg/dL), the child has hypertension, the child is exposed to tobacco, and/or the child has one or more of the following risk-increasing conditions[9]:

- *High Risk*: Type 1 and/or type 2 diabetes, kidney disease, postorthotopic heart transplant, Kawasaki disease with current coronary aneurysms

- *Moderate Risk*: Kawasaki disease with regressed coronary aneurysms, chronic inflammatory disease, HIV infection, nephrotic syndrome

Table 22-1

Acceptable, Borderline, and Abnormal Cutoff Points for Plasma Lipid, Lipoprotein, and Apolipoprotein Concentrations in Children and Adolescents

Category	Acceptable	Borderline	Abnormal
Total cholesterol (mg/dl)	< 170 (< 4.4)	170 to 199 (4.4 to 5.2)	≥ 200 (≥ 5.2)
LDL (mg/dl)	< 110 (< 2.8)	110 to 129 (2.8 to 3.3)	≥ 130 (≥ 38.4)
Non-HDL (mg/dl)	< 120 (< 3.1)	120 to 144 (3.1 to 3.7)	≥ 145 (≥ 3.8)
ApoB (mg/dl)	< 90	90 to 109	≥ 110
Triglycerides (mg/dl)	< 90 (< 1.0)	90 to 129 (1.0 to 3.3)	≥ 130 (≥ 3.4)
HDL (mg/dl)	> 45 (> 1.2)	40 to 45 (1.0 to 1.2)	< 40 (< 1.0)
ApoA-1 (mg/dl)	> 120	115 to 120	< 115

SI units are reported in parentheses.

LDL indicates low-density lipoprotein; HDL, high-density lipoprotein; ApoA-1, apolipoprotein A-1; ApoB, apolipoprotein B.

Adapted from the NHLBI's Expert panel on integrated guidelines for cardiovascular health and risk reduction in children and adolescents: summary report. *Pediatrics.* 2011;128(Suppl 5):S213-S256.

Accordingly, an abnormal lipid screening would necessitate further tracking by the medical practitioner and lipid management by a registered dietician. The NHLBI Guidelines outline recommendations following an abnormal lipid screening result. As an initial response to hyperlipidemia, unhealthy drinks should be replaced with fat-free milk or water and a limitation placed on fat and cholesterol intake (Table 22-2).[9] An energy-balanced dietary program should primarily focus on the parents for behavior modification. If improvements are not seen in lipid levels after 3 months, the guidelines suggest targeted management of hyperlipidemia.[9] In addition, if the dyslipidemic child is overweight/obese, diet management with physical activity is recommended and is most successful with family or parental involvement. If the BMI is greater than or equal to the 95th percentile of the age-sex distribution, a child should be assessed for dyslipidemia, type 2 diabetes, and hypertension. If the child is diagnosed with one or more of these comorbidities or has a BMI greater than the 97th percentile, then the child should be prescribed a program of multidisciplinary lifestyle modification focusing on physical activity and nutrition to reduce BMI. If negative for all comorbidities, the child should be given a weight loss plan involving the parents and be prescribed moderate-to-vigorous–intensity physical activity, and time spent sedentary should be decreased (see Table 22-2).[9]

Thus, the health care practitioner is confronted by several important questions when seeking to implement the NHLBI's call for universal screening, such as how universal screening can be achieved within a narrow age range at which biologic changes associated with puberty may affect the interpretation of lipid levels, how treatment of dyslipidemia in children and adolescents can be safely and effectively achieved, and whether sustained modification of the environmental risk

Table 22-2

Initial Recommendations for Hyperlipidemia Following an Abnormal Lipid Screening in Children Aged Between 9 and 11 Years

Diet Management[a]	*Focus on an energy-balanced diet; if no response after 3 months, implement lipid-specific dietary strategies*
	- Drink mostly fat-free unflavored milk
	- Replace sweetened drinks with water
	- Total fat intake should be 25% to 30% of daily kcal/EER
	- Saturated fat intake should 8% to 10% of daily kcal/EER
	- Avoid trans fat
	- Monounsaturated and polyunsaturated fat should be up to 20% of daily kcal/EER
	- Cholesterol should be limited to < 300 mg/dL
Physical Activity Management (if the child is obese)	
BMI 85th to 95th percentile	Prevent excessive weight gain by reinforcing physical activity recommendations
BMI ≥ 95th percentile	Check for T2DM and/or HTN.
	- *Without T2DM and/or HTN:* Rx for increased moderate-to-vigorous physical activity and decreased sedentary time
	- *With T2DM and/or HTN:* Refer to a multidisciplinary lifestyle program to promote weight loss
BMI ≥ 97th percentile	Refer to a multidisciplinary lifestyle program to promote weight loss

[a]Diet management for hyperlipidemia in children should be implemented under the guidance of a registered dietician.

EER indicates estimated energy requirement; HTN, hypertension; Rx, prescription; T2DM, type 2 diabetes mellitus.

Adapted from the NHLBI's Expert panel on integrated guidelines for cardiovascular health and risk reduction in children and adolescents: summary report. *Pediatrics.* 2011;128(Suppl 5):S213-S256.

factors (eg, diet, physical activity, parental smoking) is achievable, and if so, how. Nonetheless, the guidelines constitute a responsible initial approach to primordial prevention of CVD; they also provide a roadmap for screening for dysmetabolic complications early in life that will hopefully evolve into effective and fully implementable lifestyle solutions that can lead to improved health early in life and persist into adulthood as these children grow and benefit from having received early preventive interventions.

Conclusion

Extensive epidemiological evidence exists linking childhood obesity with a range of cardiovascular outcomes, including premature death. Guidelines such as those previously outlined will help pediatricians and family practitioners diagnose CVD in pediatric patients. However, the consequences of manifest CVD in childhood are serious and long lasting. CVD prevention in childhood and adolescence is almost always preferable to successful diagnosis and management of the disease. Accordingly, tackling childhood obesity and particularly addressing obesity prevention will, for the foreseeable future, remain the cornerstone in CVD prevention at any age.

References

1. Hubert HB, Feinleib M, McNamara PM, Castelli WP. Obesity as an independent risk factor for cardiovascular disease: a 26-year follow-up of participants in the Framingham Heart Study. *Circulation*. 1983;67(5):968-977.
2. Franks PW, Hanson RL, Knowler WC, Sievers ML, Bennett PH, Looker HC. Childhood obesity, other cardiovascular risk factors, and premature death. *N Engl J Med*. 2010;362(6):485-493.
3. Freedman DS, Dietz WH, Srinivasan SR, Berenson GS. The relation of overweight to cardiovascular risk factors among children and adolescents: the Bogalusa Heart Study. *Pediatrics*. 1999;103(6):1175-1182.
4. Bjørge T, Engeland A, Tverdal A, Smith GD. Body mass index in adolescence in relation to cause-specific mortality: a follow-up of 230,000 Norwegian adolescents. *Am J Epidemiol*. 2008;168(1):30-37.
5. National High Blood Pressure Education Program Working Group on High Blood Pressure in Children and Adolescents. The fourth report on the diagnosis, evaluation, and treatment of high blood pressure in children and adolescents. *Pediatrics*. 2004;114(2 Suppl 4th Report):555-576.
6. Zieske AW, Malcom GT, Strong JP. Natural history and risk factors of atherosclerosis in children and youth: the PDAY. *Pediat Pathol Mol Med*. 2002;21(2):213-237.
7. Wissler RW, Strong JP. Risk factors and progression of atherosclerosis in youth. PDAY Research Group. Pathological Determinants of Atherosclerosis in Youth. *Am J Pathol*. 1998;153(4):1023-1033.
8. Berenson GS, Srinivasan SR, Bao W, Newman WP 3rd, Tracy RE, Wattigney WA. Association between multiple cardiovascular risk factors and atherosclerosis in children and young adults. *N Engl J Med*. 1998;338(23):1650-1656.
9. Expert panel on integrated guidelines for cardiovascular health and risk reduction in children and adolescents: summary report. *Pediatrics*. 2011;128(Suppl 5):S213-S256.

Is Pediatric Obesity Associated With Cancer?

Krista Beth Highland, PhD and Kenneth P. Tercyak, PhD

Pediatricians and other primary care providers working with children, adolescents, and their families are often at the forefront of cancer prevention. In addition to providing education and counseling about the cancer risks of tobacco and alcohol use and excessive ultraviolet ray exposure from the sun and artificial sources, new data are emerging about health threats caused by being overweight and obese, including cancer. With this in mind, early intervention for cancer prevention via modification to children's diets, weights, and physical activity levels are increasingly becoming part of the national dialogue about obesity.[1]

Preventing Pediatric Cancers

Parents should be encouraged to learn steps they can take to help prevent cancer in their children. Beginning with pregnancy, pediatricians can educate expectant women about appropriate weight gain according to Institute of Medicine guidelines.[2] Although an overall pregnancy weight gain target should be kept in mind, it may useful for expectant mothers to track weight gain in weekly intervals at home using a wall calendar. Typically, normal-weight women gain 25 to 35 pounds for a single birth, with overweight and obese women gaining less. Adhering to the Institute of Medicine weight gain guidelines may help reduce the risk of childhood acute lymphocytic leukemia by as much as 12% to 38%.[3]

After birth, pediatricians can counsel new mothers to consistently breastfeed for the first 6 months of life. Parents can then introduce new foods and supplement with breastfeeding. Pediatricians and certified lactation consultants should observe breastfeeding during the first 2 weeks after birth to provide guidance and feedback. Using breast pumps may increase a mother's

Huang JS, ed. *Curbside Consultation in
Pediatric Obesity: 49 Clinical Questions* (pp 103-106).

Table 23-1
Types of Cancer Associated With Adult Obesity

- Colorectal
- Endometrial
- Esophageal
- Gastric
- Leukemia
- Liver
- Multiple myeloma

- Non-Hodgkin's lymphoma
- Ovarian
- Pancreatic
- Postmenopausal breast
- Prostate
- Renal
- Thyroid

---

ability to provide breast milk, especially if returning to work. Breast milk not only delivers antioxidants and strengthens immune functioning in offspring, but it may also reduce the risk of childhood leukemia, Hodgkin's disease, and all childhood cancers combined except leukemia and lymphoma by 15% to 35%.[4] By maintaining the recommended pregnancy weight gain and consistent breastfeeding practices, children are at a lower risk to become overweight or obese and to be affected by several types of childhood cancer.[5]

Preventing Adult Cancers

Being overweight or obese prior to adulthood has been identified as a likely contributor to several types of adult-onset cancers. For example, elevated childhood and adolescent body mass index (BMI) has been associated with renal and colon cancer in both men and women, ovarian and endometrial cancer in women, and pancreatic cancer in men.[1] Although research continues to progress, direct associations between childhood weight and adult cancer remain uncertain. One can infer that childhood obesity is associated with adult obesity, which in turn has been associated with adult-onset cancers (Table 23-1).[6] With this in mind, it is important to screen for BMI at each pediatric visit so that early intervention can occur before a child's weight becomes excessive. By intervening early and promoting healthy weight maintenance, a child's risk of future adulthood cancers may be reduced.

Pediatricians and other primary care providers are also key influences in public health campaigns to promote healthy weight and decrease future cancer risk. To help inform patients and their families in this area, it is important to adopt a standard evidence base that supports any such recommendations. This includes guidelines offered by the American Academy of Pediatrics and the American Cancer Society (Table 23-2).[7] Recommendations should address physical activity and healthy dietary practices and follow age-specific guidelines. Among school-aged youth, achieving the 60 minutes of recommended moderate to vigorous physical activity may be difficult. Toward that end, asking parents to explore a variety of age-appropriate physical activities may be beneficial to find exercises that the child enjoys, while limiting sedentary behaviors (eg, television watching, playing computer or video games) to no more than 2 hours a day. Informing parents of the daily caloric needs of children is also important but is unlikely sufficient to promote and

---

Table 23-2
American Cancer Society Guidelines on Nutrition and Physical Activity for Cancer Prevention

Achieve and Maintain a Healthy Weight Throughout Life
- Be as lean as possible throughout life without being underweight.
- Avoid excess weight gain at all ages. For those who are overweight or obese, losing even a small amount of weight has health benefits and is a good place to start.
- Get regular physical activity and limit consumption of high-calorie foods and drinks as keys to help maintain a healthy weight.

Be Physically Active
- Children and teens: Get at least 1 hour of moderate or vigorous intensity activity each day, with vigorous activity at least 3 days each week.
- Adults: Get at least 150 minutes of moderate intensity or 75 minutes of vigorous intensity activity each week (or a combination of these), preferably spread throughout the week.
- Limit sedentary behavior such as sitting, lying down, watching TV, and other forms of screen-based entertainment.

Consume a Healthy Diet, With an Emphasis on Plant-Based Foods
- Choose foods and drinks in amounts that help maintain a healthy weight.
- Limit consumption of processed meat and red meat.
- Consume at least 2.5 cups of vegetables and fruits each day.
- Choose whole grains instead of refined grain products.

---

maintain healthy behavior over time. Encourage parents to allow children to self-feed during regular structured meals, provide accessible healthy snacks and food choices (eg, fruits and vegetables), and limit calorie-dense foods that lack nutrients (eg, candy, sweetened beverages, butter, fried foods). Initial refusal does not always indicate a persistent aversion to a particular healthy food; parents should continue to offer new, healthy foods at meals. Remind parents that physical activity and healthy dietary practices not only reduce the risk of obesity throughout the lifespan but also reduce the risk of cancer in adulthood.

School-Based Cancer Prevention

Pediatricians and other child health care providers also have the potential to prevent cancer and obesity through the school setting. Intervening at schools not only increases the reach of pediatrics but may also reduce clinical hours spent coordinating health behavior changes for individual patients. Providers can serve in a variety of roles—from classroom speaker, to organizer of a school-wide assembly, to school health consultant, to school board member. When possible, join an ongoing collaboration, advisory group, or local health or education department's health promotion program to lend medical expertise in child health and development. These collaborations often draw on a wide range of lay and professional advisors, including parents, teachers, school staff, food service personnel, and community-based agency representatives that offer health education programming in schools. Goals of school involvement should include ensuring that children engage in daily moderate to vigorous exercise in physical education classes and at recesses, receive practical skills and didactics aimed at nutrition and exercise, and have ample healthy food options in the cafeteria and vending machines. This latter point can be especially effective when schools eliminate unhealthy a la carte and vending machine choices and replace them with healthier alternatives. Achieving these goals may increase the likelihood that children maintain a healthy BMI throughout childhood and into adulthood, thereby decreasing their risk of future cancers.

Conclusion

Evidence for the relationship between early-life environmental exposures and pediatric cancers is emerging. Many adult-onset cancers can be prevented or controlled by maintaining a healthy weight beginning early in childhood. Pediatricians and pediatric primary care providers should keep this information in mind and reinforce healthy lifestyle guidelines, such as those established by the Institute of Medicine, the American Academy of Pediatrics, and the American Cancer Society. Parents should be informed that maintaining a healthy weight gain during pregnancy, breastfeeding consistently for at least the first 6 months of life, and facilitating a healthy diet and physical activity pattern during childhood reduces the risk of obesity and cancer.

References

1. Fuemmeler BF, Pendzich MK, Tercyak KP. Weight, dietary behavior, and physical activity in childhood and adolescence: implications for adult cancer risk. *Obesity Facts.* 2009;2(3):179-186.
2. *Weight Gain During Pregnancy: Reexamining the Guidelines.* Washington, DC: The National Academies Press; 2009.
3. McLaughlin CC, Baptiste MS, Schymura MJ, Nasca PC, Zdeb MS. Birth weight, maternal weight, and childhood leukaemia. *Br J Cancer.* 2006;94:1738-1744.
4. Beral V, Alexander F, Appleby P. Breastfeeding and childhood cancer. *Br J Cancer.* 2000;82(5):1073-1102.
5. Mosby TT, Cosgrove M, Sarkardei S, Platt KL, Kaina B. Nutrition in adult and childhood cancer: role of carcinogens and anti-carcinogens. *Anticancer Res.* 2012;32(10):4171-4192.
6. Renehan AG, Tyson M, Egger M, Heller RF, Zwahlen M. Body-mass index and incidence of cancer: a systematic review and meta-analysis of prospective observational studies. *Lancet.* 2008;371(9612):569-578.
7. Kushi LH, Doyle C, McCullough M, et al. American Cancer Society Guidelines on nutrition and physical activity for cancer prevention: reducing the risk of cancer with healthy food choices and physical activity. *CA Cancer J Clin.* 2012;62(1):30-67.

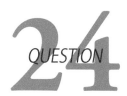

WHAT ARE THE BONE HEALTH
CONSIDERATIONS IN THE OBESE CHILD?

Heather M. Kong, MD and Sanjeev Sabharwal, MD, MPH

Obesity is a multifactorial condition that is influenced by several hormonal and metabolic factors as well as lifestyle and biomechanical changes. Not only does obesity predispose children to specific orthopedic disorders such as slipped capital femoral epiphysis and Blount disease (see Question 19), but it has implications for skeletal growth and bone health. We will explore some of these clinically relevant aspects of childhood obesity on the growing skeleton.

Advanced Bone Age

It is well known that obese children often go through puberty at an earlier age than their peers. Hormonal links exist in the pathways of estrogen with adipocytes and lectins that influence the differentiation and maturity of cartilage cells (chondrocytes) in the physis (growth plate). Because the timing of puberty is closely linked with the adolescent growth spurt, it is not surprising that obese children often have advanced skeletal maturity. With advanced puberty, obese children may begin their growth spurt earlier and thus attain skeletal maturity at an earlier age than their peers. This observation has important clinical ramifications.

For instance, growth modulation via surgery has been used to treat a variety of pediatric orthopedic disorders, such as leg-length discrepancy and angular deformities of the lower limb. This technique involves either complete (epiphysiodesis) or partial/one-sided (hemiepiphysiodesis) closure of the physis to harness and modulate the remaining growth. It is important to time this procedure accurately to avoid under- or overcorrection. The appropriate timing of this procedure is determined using history (eg, timing of menarche), physical examination (eg, Tanner staging), and established radiographic standards of skeletal growth (eg, Greulich-Pyle atlas). Although the

Huang JS, ed. *Curbside Consultation in
Pediatric Obesity: 49 Clinical Questions* (pp 107-109).
© 2014 Taylor & Francis Group

radiographic appearance of the involved physis can provide clues to the timing of closure, it is more accurate to determine skeletal (bone) age by comparing the appearance of various carpal and metacarpal bones using an anteroposterior radiograph of the child's left hand and wrist, especially during adolescence. Therefore, the phenomenon of an early growth spurt in obese children has implications for orthopedic treatments, such as guided growth for the correction of lower extremity deformities and leg-length discrepancy, as well as for counseling the family regarding the child's projected height at skeletal maturity.

Bone Mineral Density

Mixed reports exist in the literature about the effect of obesity on bone mineral density (BMD). This may be due in part to different methods for measuring and reporting BMD as areal (2-dimensional) or volumetric (3-dimensional). Some authors argue that obesity increases BMD as well as bone mineral content because of the increased mechanical stresses placed on the body. On the other hand, others have reported a higher incidence of distal extremity fractures in obese children as well as lower BMD in these patients compared with their age-matched peers. In a study examining 100 pediatric fracture patients and 100 age-matched controls, more fracture patients were overweight or obese, with lower BMD, lower bone mineral content, and higher adipose content than the controls.[1] It is likely that obese patients may have greater absolute BMD than their leaner peers but not sufficiently increased bone strength to compensate for the excessive forces applied because of their greater body mass.

Leptin has also been shown to affect BMD negatively. This adipokine stimulates the β2-adrenergic receptors on osteoblasts to inhibit trabecular bone formation. In addition, leptin acts on pluripotent mesenchymal progenitor cells to differentiate into adipocytes instead of osteoblasts. These effects have been linked to decreased cortical bone density.

Trauma

Regardless of BMD, several studies have demonstrated higher-than-expected rates of fractures among obese individuals, including children and adolescents.[2] Although this growing section of the population tends to be more sedentary and have more soft tissue "padding," which might be expected to reduce fracture risk, obese children also carry greater force on impact and tend to have gait abnormalities and impaired coordination, which may increase trauma risk. Multiple investigators have reported higher rates of distal extremity fractures and fewer femur, pelvic, and spine fractures in obese patients compared with nonobese patients.[3] This pattern has been described as the "cushion effect," whereby increased abdominal insulation has a protective effect against abdominal and pelvic injuries.[3] In addition, a biomechanical study of forearm fractures suggested that obese patients exhibit a second peak force during a fall compared with nonobese patients. Although the fracture risk is the same at the point of impact with the ground, obese patients have a greater fracture risk due to a second peak force when the patient's body weight is transmitted through the arm.

Not only does obesity increase the risk of extremity fractures, but it also influences the treatment options available for these injuries.[4] Casts and splints may be more difficult to apply appropriately and maintain because of the larger soft tissue envelope. Certain implants, such as flexible intramedullary nails for femoral shaft fractures, have a significantly higher failure rate in heavier patients, and other forms of fixation typically used in adults are thus recommended for the larger child.

The prevention of fractures and other orthopedic problems in obese children requires a multifaceted approach, including weight reduction and obesity prevention, nutritional awareness, and safety measures. Numerous organizations such as the American Academy of Orthopedic Surgeons, the Pediatric Orthopedic Society of North America, and the American Academy of Pediatrics have initiated public health campaigns to increase awareness of the effects of obesity on the musculoskeletal system. To make a sustainable impact on this growing epidemic of childhood obesity, a multipronged, collaborative approach with involvement of the family and caretakers, health care workers, and policy makers is required.

References

1. Goulding A, Jones IE, Taylor RW, Williams SM, Manning PJ. Bone mineral density and body composition in boys with distal forearm fractures: a dual-energy X-ray absorptiometry study. *J Pediatr.* 2001;139(4):509-515.
2. Gettys FK, Jackson JB, Frick SL. Obesity in pediatric orthopaedics. *Orthop Clin North Am.* 2011;42(1):95-105.
3. Arbabi S, Wahl WL, Hemmila MR, Kohoyda-Inglis C, Taheri PA, Wang SC. The cushion effect. *J Trauma.* 2003;54(6):1090-1093.
4. Lazar-Antman MA, Leet AI. Effects of obesity on pediatric fracture care and management. *J Bone Joint Surg Am.* 2012;94(9):855-861.

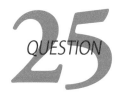

Is There Any Relationship Between Obesity and Oral Health in Children?

Raymond J. Tseng, DDS, PhD

Previous research has sought to determine whether a significant association exists between obesity and oral health (as represented by the presence of dental caries) with the assumption that obesity would be associated with a greater incidence and prevalence of dental caries in children and adolescents. As the number and scope of these dental caries studies increase, the evidence is still equivocal, with some studies showing a positive correlation and others showing no effect or a negative correlation.[1] We now know that the etiological factors that cause overweight/obesity also cause negative changes in oral health measures (but not necessarily more cavities) and that these negative effects can last into adulthood. Further, obesity-associated oral health consequences can occur earlier in life than in nonobese adolescents and last into adulthood.

The term *oral health* encompasses the health status of all hard tissues (teeth, maxilla, and mandible) and soft tissues (tongue, cheeks, gingiva, floor of mouth) that are present within the oral cavity. A healthy mouth in a child is more than just the absence of dental caries. Rather, it includes the presence of healthy and normal growth and development of the teeth and other orofacial structures. Thus, to answer the question of whether any relationship exists between obesity and oral health, one should look beyond the most obvious issue of the development of dental caries to alterations in long-term dentofacial growth and development, changes in the health status of the gingiva and periodontium, and increased risk for gingivitis or periodontal disease.

Many factors contribute to the development of childhood overweight and obesity. A sedentary lifestyle, lack of physical activity, excessive consumption of sugar-sweetened beverages (SSB), and an unbalanced diet composed of calorie-dense, nutrient-poor foods are all factors that lead to obesity. In addition, children of racial/ethnic minorities, as well as those from families with low socioeconomic status, disproportionately suffer from higher rates of childhood overweight and obesity.[2,3] Irrespective of weight status, some of these demographic and social factors are

Huang JS, ed. *Curbside Consultation in Pediatric Obesity: 49 Clinical Questions* (pp 111-114).
© 2014 Taylor & Francis Group

also positively associated with negative oral health outcomes. Low socioeconomic status, being a member of a racial minority, lack of a college education, and excessive consumption of SSB are all factors that have been linked with poor oral health and increased caries risk. Thus, it is not necessarily overweight/obesity that causes increases in dental caries. Rather, the factors linked with obesity may demonstrate main associations with poor oral health.[2]

Obesity itself is known to cause changes in nearly every physiological system and biological process in the body. These effects include an acceleration of growth and development (as indicated by an earlier onset of puberty), changes in inflammation, and alterations in immune function.[3] Changes in these processes also alter oral health outcomes (not necessarily dental caries) that depend on these processes.

A review of the medical and social history of the child and family, and questions about lifestyle, diet, and nutrition may indicate several risk factors for obesity-associated oral health consequences in infants and children. These findings may include parents who themselves are overweight or obese, excessive consumption of juice or other SSB at an early age, grazing on foods that contain cariogenic fermentable carbohydrates, and going to sleep with a bottle filled with juice or other SSB. Listed below are clinical symptoms that may present in children during well-child visits. All of these symptoms are rooted in the premise that the longer teeth are in the mouth and the more they are exposed to cariogenic foods/beverages, the faster they will decay and the earlier a child will need dental restorations.

Accelerated Eruption of Teeth

Obesity is associated with a general acceleration in maturation and an earlier onset of puberty.[4] This acceleration also applies to the formation and eruption of permanent teeth. Accelerated eruption could manifest as an earlier time point of initial tooth eruption into the mouth and/or a shortened duration of time needed for each tooth to fully erupt. A recent study of children and adolescents showed that increased body mass index (BMI) percentile was associated with accelerated dental development of the permanent teeth.[5,6] The clinical implication is that if teeth erupt into the mouth at an earlier age, they are exposed to a cariogenic environment for a longer period of time and thus are more likely to require restorations at an earlier age. Accelerated growth and development could also potentially affect primary teeth, although more studies are needed at this time. The normal eruption time of primary teeth occurs between 6 and 33 months. For infants and children, the combination of early eruption of primary teeth, prolonged exposure to a cariogenic environment, and low efficacy of oral hygiene will likely result in a greater number of dental caries with increased severity. In infants and children, every preventive effort should be made to minimize the need for dental treatment early in life.

Earlier Onset and Greater Severity of Demineralization and Dental Caries

An obesogenic diet is generally higher in sugar and fermentable carbohydrates, which is directly related to the development of dental caries. In addition, foods/beverages that are grazed on throughout the day have greater cariogenic potential than if they were consumed only at meal-times. In infants and children, increased exposure to SSB and other cariogenic foods leads to the buildup of bacteria and plaque and results in demineralization and subsequently dental caries. This is especially true in primary teeth, which have thinner enamel and less protection against cariogenic bacteria than their permanent dentition counterparts. The relationship between obesity and dental caries is equivocal.[1] It is influenced by demographic, lifestyle, and other developmental/physiological factors. In children with a highly cariogenic diet and poor oral hygiene, we would expect to see a higher incidence of caries, irrespective of weight status. A thorough analysis of all risk factors for dental caries is prudent in overweight and obese children.

Accelerated Breakdown of Hypoplastic Teeth

Hypoplastic teeth are characterized by abnormal formation of the teeth, resulting in weakened enamel, increased fracture, and breakdown of the teeth. Obesity itself is not identified as a risk factor for the presence of hypoplastic teeth. Because of the lack of protection and structural integrity, hypoplastic teeth are especially prone to breakdown, more so than teeth that have normal enamel and dentin. Hypoplastic primary molars can erupt into the mouth as early as 13 months. An obesogenic diet could lead to accelerated breakdown of these teeth, resulting in placement of stainless steel crowns and possible pulpotomies, or "baby root canals." In severe cases, an obesogenic diet and a lack of early dental care may result in the need for extraction of primary teeth at an early age, which has subsequent consequences for craniofacial growth and development, speech development, diet and nutrition, a child's ability to thrive, and social development.

Increased Risk and Earlier Onset for Gingivitis and Periodontal Disease

Obesity is associated with alterations in inflammation.[7] The development of obesity has also been associated with a higher incidence and earlier age of onset of several obesity-related pathologies and conditions, such as diabetes and hypertension.[8] Consistent with this, obesity is associated with a greater severity of gingivitis in overweight/obese adolescents.[9] Chronic gingivitis subsequently gives rise to an earlier onset of periodontal disease (PD) in adolescents and young adults, once thought to be a disease of older adults.[9] Specifically, current research now shows that the incidence of PD is increasing in young adults, and the presence of PD risk factors is on the rise in adolescents. PD is characterized by an inflammation of the gingival and increased probing pocket depth, indicative of bone resorption surrounding the permanent dentition in both adolescents and adults.[9,10]

For overweight or obese children, prevention of these oral health consequences is possible through early identification of risk factors, application of preventive fluoride varnishes, and referral to knowledgeable dental providers who are comfortable working with children. The pediatrician can perform the following tasks.

KEEP A LIST OF GENERAL AND PEDIATRIC DENTISTS WHO SEE CHILDREN AT AGE 1 YEAR TO ESTABLISH A DENTAL HOME

Encourage parents to have their child visit a knowledgeable general or pediatric dentist by the age of 1 year. These visits are more than meet-and-greet appointments. The right dental provider can provide the following:

- A thorough dental examination to identify hypoplastic teeth and other conditions that increase the risk of development of dental caries
- Anticipatory guidance regarding safe consumption habits of foods and beverages to minimize caries risk and the risk of early development of childhood overweight or obesity (working in conjunction with the child's pediatrician)

- Information about the right timing and technique of using a fluoridated toothpaste to strengthen enamel and prevent cavities

- Acclimation for the baby in the dental office. Although a 1-year-old child may engage in age-appropriate crying, children who establish a dental home early will generally become acclimated to dental visits more quickly, have fewer caries, and have a better dental experience if restorative services are required.[11,12]

APPLY FLUORIDE VARNISH TO TEETH

Fluoride varnish can be quickly and safely applied at well-child visits and has been shown to significantly reduce the development of dental caries.[13] In children who are prone to obesity and who may consume a highly cariogenic diet, regular application of fluoride varnish every 6 months until the child has established a dental home is a safe and effective way to minimize the risk of dental caries.

SHARE BODY MASS INDEX DATA

As childhood obesity becomes more prevalent, you may find pediatric dentists who record height and weight data at regular intervals, which allows the opportunity to collect longitudinal height, weight, and BMI percentile information. Establishing a good relationship with these dentists can help with monitoring weight status and can be used collaboratively by pediatric health care providers and dentists alike to identify the development of obesity.

References

1. Kantovitz KR, Pascon FM, Rontani RM, Gavião MB. Obesity and dental caries—a systematic review. *Oral Health Prev Dent*. 2006;4(2):137-144.
2. Spiegel KA, Palmer CA. Childhood dental caries and childhood obesity. Different problems with overlapping causes. *Am J Dent*. 2012;25(1):59-64.
3. Dietz WH. Health consequences of obesity in youth: childhood predictors of adult disease. *Pediatrics*. 1998;101(3 Pt 2):518-525.
4. Cheng G, Buyken AE, Shi L, et al. Beyond overweight: nutrition as an important lifestyle factor influencing timing of puberty. *Nutr Rev*. 2012;70(3):133-152.
5. Mack KB, Phillips C, Jain N, Koroluk LD. Relationship between body mass index percentile and skeletal maturation and dental development in orthodontic patients. *Am J Orthod Dentofacial Orthop*. 2013;142(2):228-234.
6. Hilgers KK, Akridge M, Scheetz JP, Kinane DE. Childhood obesity and dental development. *Pediatr Dent*. 2006;28(1):18-22.
7. Tran B, Oliver S, Rosa J, Galassetti P. Aspects of inflammation and oxidative stress in pediatric obesity and type 1 diabetes: an overview of ten years of studies. *Exp Diabetes Res*. 2012;2012:683680.
8. Herouvi D, Karanasios E, Karayianni C, Karavanaki K. Cardiovascular disease in childhood: the role of obesity. *Eur J Pediatr*. 2013;172(6):721-732.
9. Fadel HT, Pliaki A, Gronowitz E, et al. Clinical and biological indicators of dental caries and periodontal disease in adolescents with or without obesity [published online ahead of print March 21, 2013]. *Clin Oral Investig*.
10. Chaffee BW, Weston SJ. Association between chronic periodontal disease and obesity: a systematic review and meta-analysis. *J Periodontol*. 2010;81(12):1708-1724.
11. Lee JY, Bowens TJ, Savage MF, Vann WF Jr. Examining the cost-effectiveness of early dental visits. *Pediatr Dent*. 2006;28(2):102-105.
12. Savage MF, Lee JY, Kotch JB, Vann WF Jr. Early preventive dental visits: effects on subsequent utilization and costs. *Pediatrics*. 2004;114(4):e418-e423.
13. Miller EK, Vann WF Jr. The use of fluoride varnish in children: a critical review with treatment recommendations. *J Clin Pediatr Dent*. 2008;32(4):259-264.

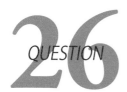

SOME OF MY OBESE PATIENTS COMPLAIN
ABOUT BEING BULLIED. WHAT SHOULD I SAY TO THESE
PATIENTS AND FAMILIES? WHAT IS MY RESPONSIBILITY?

Joseph A. Skelton, MD, MS and Dara Garner-Edwards, MSW, LCSW

Bullying is serious and should not be taken lightly, and in the lives of overweight and obese children, it appears to be even more problematic. Obese children are more likely to be bullied, regardless of other social or academic factors.[1] School-aged children have much higher odds of being bullied if they are overweight or obese.[2] In addition to being bullied, these children are more likely to be victims of aggression or loss of friendships; targets of rumors and lies; or prone to name calling, teasing, hitting, and kicking.[2] Unfortunately, obese children can also become the perpetrators themselves, with older adolescents (aged 15 to 16 years) being more likely to bully their normal-weight classmates. Bullying can affect the self-esteem and well-being of children, has the potential to inflict long-lasting physical and emotional harm, and could be a contributor to concerns of children's quality of life, which is known to be affected by weight.[3]

Physicians should differentiate between teasing and bullying in planning how to best help their patients. Differences between teasing and bullying can seem small, but their impact is not, and additional effort and time is needed by the physician to determine what is occurring in the child's life. Furthermore, interventions differ according to whether a child is the receiver or perpetrator of teasing versus bullying. Teasing is a broader term that includes a continuum of actions from friendly banter between friends to hostility and bullying.[4] Parents and adults rarely hear of mild teasing because it often does not upset the child. However, this teasing can become hurtful and is moderated by the child's response, which can vary widely depending on the child and situation. This calls attention to a particular difficulty related to the assessment of teasing because one child may be upset, hurt, or embarrassed by the teasing and others may not. Parents, teachers, and physicians should be sensitive of this fact when assessing an incident. Lastly, teasing can become hostile to the point where it is bullying and inflicting emotional distress or even physical harm on a child.

Huang JS, ed. Curbside Consultation in
Pediatric Obesity: 49 Clinical Questions (pp 115-119).
© 2014 Taylor & Francis Group

Bullying, as defined by experts and researchers, is "when [a child] is exposed, repeatedly and over time, to negative actions on the part of one or more other [children]."[5(p9)] Negative actions can be carried out by physical contact, words, making faces or dirty gestures, or intentional exclusion from a group.[5] An additional criterion of bullying is "an imbalance in strength (an asymmetric power relationship) where the student who is exposed to the negative actions has difficulty defending him- or herself."[5(p10)] The imbalance of power and strength and the child's inability or difficulty in defending himself or herself are what makes this situation potentially serious, necessitating support from adults. The Centers for Disease Control (CDC) has identified bullying as a public health concern, identifying key components of bullying as the following:

- Attack or intimidation with the Intention to cause fear, distress, or harm

- A real or perceived imbalance of power between the bully and the victim

- Repeated attacks or intimidation between the same children over time

Similarly to the CDC, the American Academy of Pediatrics addresses bullying, not from a self-esteem or emotional perspective, but from one of youth violence prevention.[6] They define bullying as "a form of aggression in which one or more children repeatedly and intentionally intimidate, harass, or physically harm a victim who is perceived as unable to defend herself or himself."[6(p395)]

Differentiating between teasing and bullying is important. Children can learn skills to manage teasing and therefore lessen the impact it has on them. In bullying, the child feels powerless to stop the situation, and thus the situation requires adult intervention. Following Freedman's concept of teasing and bullying as parts of a single continuum,[4] bullying can begin as teasing and become more and more aggressive so that the child develops feelings of powerlessness. The distinguishing factor that differentiates teasing behavior from bullying is the child's perception of vulnerability and the repetitive and harmful nature of the behavior. We can trust the child's perception as our definition of whether the behavior is teasing or bullying.

What is your responsibility? For teasing, physicians can rely on the family and school to respond. The child should receive your support and be encouraged to access school or family support depending on that child's nature and specific needs. School staff can assist a child being teased with learning skills to identify their own emotional response and practice different methods of responding to the teasing. Table 26-1 is an example of strategies that can be taught to students experiencing teasing. Children can select approaches that fit their personality and specific situations. To keep the learning simple, the child can select 2 or 3 possible approaches and practice them with an adult prior to using them with the teaser. These strategies build coping skills and empower the child with tools for responding to teasing. Although any particular response can help reduce the teasing or give the child more confidence during the exchange, adults must understand that using the responses is not a guarantee that teasing will end. The goal of teaching such skills is to build the child's confidence in applying effective techniques so that even when the child cannot control the teaser's behavior, he or she can better control his or her own reaction and coping.

What about bullying? Bullying requires adult intervention. The recipient child perceives that he or she cannot stop the bully's behavior and therefore needs assistance. As physicians, we can trust the child's perception and act to protect the child who feels vulnerable. First, if parents and caregivers are not aware of the bullying, take steps to alert them. If the child or adolescent told you in confidence, include the child in a disclosure to the parents. Second, a key resource in instances of bullying is the child's school, which often has strong programs to respond to bullying situations and will take this seriously. It is appropriate for you, someone in your office such as a nurse, or the parent to alert the child's teacher, school counselor, school social worker, or principal. If performed by you or your office, this communication requires the consent of the family unless the child is in immediate danger. Once the school staff is aware, they can guide the response within the school to support the student and address the bullying. If you are concerned the parents may not call the

Table 26-1
Skills to Teach Children Who Are Being Teased

Technique	Explanation
Self-talk	Child can say positive things in his or her head to counter hurtful teasing. "I can handle this." "Who cares what Bobby says?" Child can also focus on own positive traits.
Ignoring	Rather than crying or screaming, act unaffected. Do not look at or respond to the tease. OK to walk away. Lack of response reduces teaser's power and impact.
The "I" message	Child learns to politely express own feelings. "I feel _____ when _____ and I would like you to stop." This can confuse the teaser.
Visualization	Child can imagine a force field around self that repels the mean words or other positive image of protection during the teasing. This allows child not to accept the hurtful statements.
Turning the tease around	Reframing the tease. Teaser says, "That shirt makes you look big as a house!" Child responds, "Thanks for noticing my style!"
Agreeing with the teaser	Agree with facts. Teaser says, "You are eating the whole pizza!" Child says, "Pizza is my favorite food." Agreeing can remove need to hide the taunted trait.
"So?"	This allows child to appear unaffected. Very simple and useful.
Complimenting the teaser	When child is teased about walking slowly to class, child can say, "You are a faster walker and will get to class first again today."
Humor	Laughing or making a joke can take the tension out of the situation for both child and teaser.

Adapted from Freedman J. *Easing the Teasing*. Chicago, IL: Contemporary Books; 2002.

school or the child may convince them not to, follow through with calling the school yourself to make sure it is being addressed.

For the child who is bullying others, similar approaches can beneficial. Most children bully for attention, for acceptance from peers, or to imitate others, and attempts can be made to identify what is behind the child's behavior. Parents should discuss the issue with the child in a respectful manner, taking care not to shame him or her. The family will need the support of the school, particularly teachers and school counselors, to change the behavior. If the bullying continues, therapists and counselors can provide further guidance and support in working with the child and family.

Providing support and guidance to parents is also important. Taking the time to explain the difference between teasing and bullying to parents can help them understand the situation and potential problems that could arise. It is important that they understand that bullying requires adult intervention and is not simply "kids being kids." This is also a time to make them aware of the school as a resource, even beyond teachers and principals. The following include other important issues to consider:

- *Safety*: Take time to assess the child's safety. Ask questions about what the bully is doing to the child to determine if verbal and/or physical abuse are factors. If the abuse is physical, assess injuries and consider the child's safety as an urgent concern. If the child is feeling hopeless about the bullying, it is appropriate to ask the child if self-harm or revenge has been considered (using words like, "You are feeling so hopeless about what is happening; have you thought of hurting yourself? Have you thought of hurting anyone else?"). If the child is having thoughts of self-harm or harm to others, further mental health assessment is warranted.

- *Severity*: Bullying can be more intimidating when the child feels isolated. Isolation can be physical or social. If the child is on a school bus, limited options exist for adult assistance, and the bully has more leeway for hostility. If the child is alone in the environment where the teasing occurs, the child is also more vulnerable. If the child lacks friends in general, any ridicule can be perceived as harmful. Isolation, either physical or social, speaks to the need for adult intervention to prevent escalation or harm.

- *Cyber-bullying*: When bullying occurs via electronic outlets like telephones, texting, e-mail, or social media, it is called *cyber-bullying*. Cyber-bullying is a significant problem as evidenced by several high-profile tragedies in the past few years. This form of bullying is not limited to school or social relationships because the Internet allows for children to interact across schools or even greater distances. If peers at school are involved, the child's teacher or principal is an appropriate resource. Sometimes, if the bullying does not occur during hours where the child is in class, school administrators may be hesitant to get involved, and parents may need support in communicating the seriousness to the school. Principals and administrators can be a resource if a student at another school is the perpetrator by contacting the principal at that school. If the school is not involved, this type of bullying requires a different response. Depending on the seriousness or threat involved, parents can still approach the school for assistance, report the incident to managers of the website or social media outlet, which typically have active channels for reporting abuse, or even report to local law enforcement. Parents can also have numbers blocked through their cellular phone service providers to prevent their child from receiving threatening or menacing texts or calls, and the same intervention can be performed with Web-based blogs and e-mail.

Physicians can be a significant resource to parents, children, and families who are experiencing bullying. The first step is to determine if the child is experiencing teasing and its effect or if he or she is dealing with the more serious issue of bullying. If bullying is involved, a potential exists for significant stress in the life of the child as well as a potential for violence, thus necessitating adult intervention. Parents and children may also benefit from understanding the differences between teasing and bullying. Physicians can support parents in addressing the problem by encouraging them to contact school administrators and/or even advocate themselves for the child by contacting the school directly.

Acknowledgment

The authors would like to thank Amy Mooney for her assistance.

References

1. Lumeng JC, Forrest P, Appugliese DP, Kaciroti N, Corwyn RF, Bradley RH. Weight status as a predictor of being bullied in third through sixth grades. *Pediatrics*. 2010;125(6):e1301-e1307.
2. Janssen I, Craig WM, Boyce WF, Pickett W. Associations between overweight and obesity with bullying behaviors in school-aged children. *Pediatrics*. 2004;113(5):1187-1194.
3. Schwimmer JB, Burwinkle TM, Varni JW. Health-related quality of life of severely obese children and adolescents. *JAMA*. 2003;289(14):1813-1819.
4. Freedman J. *Easing the Teasing*. Chicago, IL: Contemporary Books; 2002.
5. Olweus D. *Bullying at School: What We Know and What We Can Do*. Cambridge, MA: Blackwell Publishers Ltd; 1993.
6. Committee on Injury, Violence, and Poison Prevention. Policy statement—Role of the pediatrician in youth violence prevention. *Pediatrics*. 2009;124(1):393-402.

Suggested Readings

American Academy of Child and Adolescent Psychiatry. Bullying Resource Center. http://www.aacap.org/AACAP/Families_and_Youth/Resource_Centers/Bullying_Resource_Center/Home.aspx. Updated August 2012. Accessed March 5, 2014.

Centers for Disease Control and Prevention. Understanding Bullying Fact Sheet. 2012. http://www.cdc.gov/ViolencePrevention/pdf/BullyingFactsheet2012-a.pdf. Accessed March 5, 2014.

National Crime Prevention Council. http://www.ncpc.org. Accessed March 5, 2014.

US Department of Health and Human Services. http://www.stopbullying.gov. Accessed March 5, 2014.

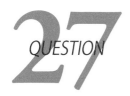

QUESTION 27

ARE QUALITY OF LIFE AND SELF-ESTEEM ALTERED IN OBESE CHILDREN? ARE PSYCHIATRIC DISORDERS MORE COMMON IN OBESE CHILDREN?

Margarita D. Tsiros, PhD and Alison M. Coates, PhD

Understanding how obesity influences psychosocial and emotional wellness in children is an essential component in the effective management of the obese child, and it allows identification of potential barriers to treatment uptake.[1] Of upmost importance is the impact on children's quality of life—that is, their satisfaction and enjoyment relating to their own physical, mental, and social well-being. Tied in with this are factors such as children's self-esteem (ie, their sense of self-worth) and whether they have any psychiatric disorders.

It is well known that children with obesity have lower global health-related quality of life (HRQoL) than their healthy-weight peers, with the most notable impairments in their physical and psychosocial functioning.[1-3] In fact, HRQoL starts to suffer as soon as children are above their ideal weight, well before they reach the threshold for obesity.[2,3] Upon closer inspection, effects on psychosocial HRQoL may be largely due to particular problems with social functioning, whereas impacts on emotional functioning are less obvious and are clouded by factors such as child age and method of reporting (ie, self-report versus parent-proxy reports).[1,2]

The self-esteem literature paints a similar picture, with strong evidence that obesity is linked with lower global self-esteem in children.[1] Subdomains of self-esteem hold a similar pattern to HRQoL research, in part due to overlap between what currently available tools actually measure, suggesting that athletic/physical competence and perceptions of physical appearance are most strongly affected, along with social functioning and acceptance. However, the interplay between obesity and self-esteem is complex and probably reciprocal given longitudinal evidence that lower global self-esteem increases the odds of developing overweight/obesity later in childhood/adolescence.[4]

Improvements in global HRQoL and self-esteem may result following weight loss, with physical and social subdomain gains most likely to occur (eg, functioning, competence, appearance and

Huang JS, ed. *Curbside Consultation in*
Pediatric Obesity: 49 Clinical Questions (pp 121-126).
© 2014 Taylor & Francis Group

acceptance).[1,2] However, saying that improving children's self-regard and HRQoL is simply a matter of losing weight would be misleading, particularly given the minimal evidence of a continuous relationship between reductions in weight status and improvements in HRQoL/self-esteem scores.[1,2] In truth, the relationships between obesity and HRQoL/self-esteem are likely to be exceedingly complex, requiring further research.

Psychological complications faced by obese youth are becoming increasingly recognized, although prevalence rates are hard to determine because of differences in definitions. United States statistics[5] using the *Diagnostic and Statistical Manual of Mental Disorders*[6] suggest that the most common psychiatric disorders experienced by 8- to 15-year-olds are attention deficit/hyperactivity disorder, followed by mood disorders, conduct disorder, panic disorder or generalized anxiety disorder, and eating disorders. Rates of these psychiatric diagnoses appear to be greater in children who are overweight or have obesity-related health conditions relative to children with other chronic health conditions.[7]

Youths seeking treatment for their obesity appear to be more prone to developing psychiatric disorders, although this could reflect better screening by practitioners compared with community populations. The presence of such complications may create a negative cycle, compounding weight gain and reducing success with weight management; hence, it is important to identify and manage such conditions carefully. A 2-tiered approach is recommended. In general practice settings, a discussion with both the child and parent/caregiver should inquire into the HRQoL and psychological functioning of all overweight and obese children. Questions should address physical, social, emotional, and school function life domains and address both depression and anxiety.[8] Those children identified with a body mass index >99% or those presenting for obesity management should also complete a behavior assessment. A range of useful tools is summarized in Table 27-1.

Although a range of psychological/psychiatric disorders are associated with obesity in childhood and adolescence, the strength of these associations is not as great as one might think and appears to be affected by other factors like sex, age, socioeconomic status, stigma, teasing, and maternal mental health.[8] The strength of these associations can be grouped as either small-to-moderate or negligible-to-small associations (Table 27-2). Many of these disorders affect each other, with severity and prevalence increasing dramatically when factors such as teasing and/or obesity stigma are present. These weak associations suggest that certain children may be resilient to developing psychological conditions. Future research should focus on identifying what protective factors help develop resilience.

It is important to acknowledge that psychiatric comorbidities may be a cause or consequence of childhood and adolescent obesity, or they may share common causative factors.[7] Some evidence exists that depression in childhood is a predictor of obesity, but less evidence exists that pediatric obesity predicts depression.[8] However, such relationships between obesity and other psychiatric conditions are less clear[4] and require ongoing research.

Interventions to improve the weight status of obese children are paramount, but considering the psychological well-being of the child is just as important because it not only contributes to the child's readiness and capacity to engage in management but also to his or her long-term outcome. Unlike many of the physical/health morbidities linked with obesity, the risk of negative well-being and self-worth are immediate. Although lifestyle approaches such as improving diet, physical activity, and sedentary behavior are the cornerstone of weight management, incorporating cognitive and/or behavioral strategies and engaging family and peer support have been shown to improve treatment outcomes. Therefore, children may benefit from such combined interventions incorporating psychological approaches (eg, cognitive and behavioral strategies) specifically targeted at improving physical and social functioning/self-regard. This must be differentiated from a child with a suspected psychiatric disorder, who must be referred for appropriate individualized management by a psychiatrist.

Table 27-1

Summary of Tools Commonly Used to Assess Psychological Complications in Children

Tool	Questionnaire Details	Parent-Proxy/Child Self-Reported	Target Demographic	Psychometric Properties of Tools
Sizing Them Up[a] http://www.cincinnatichildrens.org/research/divisions/c/adherence/labs/modi/hrqol/sizing/default/	22 item questionnaire 6 subscales: 1. Emotional functioning 2. Physical functioning 3. Teasing/marginalization 4. Positive social attributes 5. Mealtime challenges 6. School functioning	Parent-proxy report	Children aged 5 to 18 years	Internal consistency coefficients α = 0.59 to 0.91. Test-retest reliability = 0.57 to 0.80.
Sizing Me Up[a] http://www.cincinnatichildrens.org/research/divisions/c/adherence/labs/modi/hrqol/sizing/default/	22-item questionnaire 5 subscales: 1. Emotional functioning 2. Physical functioning 3. Social avoidance 4. Positive social attributes 5. Teasing/marginalization	Child self-report	Children aged 5 to 13 years	Internal consistency coefficients α = 0.68 to 0.85. Test-retest reliability = 0.53 to 0.78.
Lifestyle Behavior Checklist[a] http://informahealthcare.com/doi/abs/10.3109/17477160902811199?journalCode=jpo	26-item weight-related problem behaviors 2 subscales: 1. Problem scale (extent of problems) 2. Confidence scale (parents' confidence in dealing with these problems)	Parent-proxy report	Children aged 4 to 11 years	Internal consistency coefficients α = 0.87 to 0.95 and moderate test-retest stability

(continued)

Table 27-1 (continued)

Summary of Tools Commonly Used to Assess Psychological Complications in Children

Tool	Questionnaire Details	Parent-Proxy/Child Self-Reported	Target Demographic	Psychometric Properties of Tools
Impact of Weight on Quality of Life-Kids (IWQOL-Kids)[a] http://www. qualityoflifeconsulting. com/iwqol-kids.html	27-item questionnaire 4 subscales: 1. Physical comfort 2. Emotional (body esteem) 3. Social life 4. Family relations	Child self-report and parent-proxy versions available	Children aged 11 to 19 years	High internal consistency (ranging from $\alpha = 0.88$ to 0.95 for scales, and $=0.96$ for total score)
Youth Quality-of-Life Instrument–Weight module (YQOL-W)[a] http://depts.washington. edu/seaqol/YQOL-W	21 weight-specific item questionnaire 3 subscales: 1. Self (emotional) 2. Social 3. Environment	Child self-report	Children aged 11 to 18 years	Test-retest intraclass correlation coefficients $=0.73$ for Social, 0.71 for Self, 0.73 for Environment, and 0.77 for the 1-factor model.
Pediatric Quality of Life Inventory (PedsQL 4.0) http://www.pedsql.org/ about_pedsql.html	23-item questionnaire 4 subscales: 1. Physical 2. Emotional 3. Social 4. School functioning	Child self-report and parent-proxy versions available	Children aged 4 to 11 years	Reliability coefficients Total scale score$=0.88$ (child self-report) and 0.90 (parent proxy-report)

(continued)

Table 27-1 (continued)

Summary of Tools Commonly Used to Assess Psychological Complications in Children

Tool	Questionnaire Details	Parent-Proxy/Child Self-Reported	Target Demographic	Psychometric Properties of Tools
Behavior Assessment System for Children (BASC-2)[b]	Broad-based measures of psychological well-being 5 scales: 1. Teacher Rating Scales (TRS) 2. Parent Rating Scales (PRS) 3. Self-Report of Personality (SRP) 4. Structured Developmental History (SDH) form 5. Student Observation System (SOS)	Child self-report, parent- proxy and teacher forms to complete	Children aged 2 to 21 years	Moderate-to-good reliability and validity. Scales and composites have high internal consistency (α = 0.80 with children and 0.90 with adolescents) and test-retest reliability.
The Achenbach Child Behaviour Checklist (CBCL)[b]	Broad-based measures of behavioral and emotional problems 113-item questionnaire 8 syndrome scales: 1. Anxious/depressed 2. Depressed 3. Somatic complaints 4. Social problems 5. Thought problems 6. Attention problems 7. Rule-breaking behavior 8. Aggressive behavior	Child self-report	Children aged 6 to 18 years	Reliability coefficients ranged from 0.71 to 0.89.

[a]Obesity-specific quality-of-life screening tools. [b]These tools are recommended for assessment of children with a body mass index sex-and-age matched > 99% or those presenting for obesity management.

Table 27-2

Psychological Complications Associated With Obesity in Children and Adolescents[a]

Small-to-moderate[a] associations (r value = 0.1 to 0.5)	Negligible-to-small[a] associations (r value > 0.1)
Body dissatisfaction	Low self-esteem
Symptoms of depression	Clinically significant depression
Loss of control eating	Full syndrome eating disorders
Extreme or unhealthy weight control behaviors	Suicide
Impaired social relationships	
Stigma (related to obesity)	
Impaired HRQoL	
Anxiety disorders	

[a]Mediators of these relationships: demographic variables (age, sex, race, ethnicity, socioeconomic status), stigma, teasing and maternal mental health.

Adapted from Vander Wal JS, Mitchell ER. Psychological complications of pediatric obesity. *Pediatr Clin North Am.* 2011;58(6):1393-1401.

As a final and possibly obvious point, clinicians should always undertake assessments of a child's well-being, self-esteem, and psychological state before, during, and after any weight-management intervention. Many generic and obesity-specific tools exist, along with a number of systematic reviews to assist clinicians to select the most appropriate tools for their clinical practice. Commonly used tools to evaluate psychological complications in obese children and adolescents are listed in Table 27-1.

References

1. Griffiths LJ, Parsons TJ, Hill AJ. Self-esteem and quality of life in obese children and adolescents: a systematic review. *Int J Pediatr Obes.* 2010;5(4):282-304.
2. Tsiros MD, Olds T, Buckley JD, et al. Health-related quality of life in obese children and adolescents. *Int J Obes (Lond).* 2009;33(4):387-400.
3. Ul-Haq Z, Mackay DF, Fenwick E, Pell JP. Meta-analysis of the association between body mass index and health-related quality of life among children and adolescents, assessed using the pediatric quality of life inventory index. *J Pediatr.* 2013;162(2):280-286.
4. Incledon E, Wake M, Hay M. Psychological predictors of adiposity: systematic review of longitudinal studies. *Int J Pediatr Obes.* 2011;6(2-2):e1-e11.
5. Merikangas KR, He JP, Brody D, Fisher PW, Bourdon K, Koretz DS. Prevalence and treatment of mental disorders among US children in the 2001-2004 NHANES. *Pediatrics.* 2010;125(1):75-81.
6. American Psychiatric Association. Diagnostic and statistical manual of mental disorders (DSM-IV-TR). 4th ed. Washington DC; 2000.
7. Kalarchian MA, Marcus MD. Psychiatric comorbidity of childhood obesity. *Int Rev Psychiatry.* 2012;24(3):241-246.
8. Vander Wal JS, Mitchell ER. Psychological complications of pediatric obesity. *Pediatr Clin North Am.* 2011;58(6):1393-1401.

QUESTION 28

DOES PEDIATRIC OBESITY PREDICT ADULT OBESITY? DOES BEING OVERWEIGHT OR OBESE AS A CHILD REDUCE ONE'S LIFESPAN EXPECTANCY?

Lee Ann E. Conard, RPh, DO, MPH and Frank M. Biro, MD

Most clinicians use body mass index (BMI) as a measure of the degree of obesity. Determination of BMI is fairly straightforward, calculated easily from height and weight (BMI = weight/height^2, in kilograms and meters; if using pounds and inches, weight × 703/height^2). The Centers for Disease Control also has a calculator online at http://www.cdc.gov/healthyweight/assessing/bmi/adult_bmi/english_bmi_calculator/bmi_calculator.html.

BMI difference between individuals captures the majority of variation in adiposity, but is also influenced by muscle mass, sex, age, and fitness. In addition, BMI does not capture body fat distribution, which is determined more accurately by waist-to-height ratio.[1] Despite these limitations, BMI still serves a useful approach to categorizing degrees of obesity and subsequent risks for morbidity and mortality. The World Health Organization published a classification of adult obesity based on BMI: a BMI of 25.0 to 29.9 kg/m^2 represents overweight, 30.0 to 34.9 kg/m^2 represents class I obesity, 35.0 to 39.9 kg/m^2 represents class II obesity, and 40.0 kg/m^2 or more represents class III obesity. In children, weight status is classified according to BMI percentiles with regard to age and sex (see Question 1).

When we as clinicians speak with patients and parents about obesity, parents are often surprised that we perceive that their child is overweight/obese, and they believe that their child just needs time to "lose their baby fat," even when the patient is an adolescent. Nevertheless, several studies show that obese children are more likely to become obese adults. A meta-analysis examined BMI tracking in 48 international cohort studies with a mean follow-up of 14.6 years and found a high degree of body composition tracking, as measured by BMI. The authors noted that the observed tracking estimates implied a low likelihood of spontaneous weight changes among individuals not under weight loss treatment.[2] In a similar review, persistence of overweight rose with an increasing level of overweight and increasing age.[3]

Huang JS, ed. *Curbside Consultation in Pediatric Obesity: 49 Clinical Questions* (pp 127-129).
© 2014 Taylor & Francis Group

Parents of overweight children are often overweight themselves and tell us that other family members are overweight, and yet they do not seem to understand why we are worried about their child's weight. To address this gap, we clinicians often talk with parents about morbidity and mortality associated with obesity. We discuss the consequences of childhood and adolescent obesity, including earlier puberty and menarche in girls, type 2 diabetes and increased incidence of metabolic syndrome in youth and adults, polycystic ovarian syndrome (PCOS), and obesity in adulthood. Obese adults are at higher risk for obesity-related conditions, such as type 2 diabetes, osteoarthritis, cardiovascular disease, ischemic stroke, and several specific types of cancer. Of note, the adult cardiovascular risks for obese children track along the risks for obese adults, with some interesting variances noted in 3 recent longitudinal studies. Cardiovascular risk factors in children were clustered and found to track across childhood into adolescence. These findings were more prominent when stratified by fitness but not when stratified by degree of fatness.[4] BMI in the child or adolescent tracked along cardiovascular risks of the adult except in early childhood, where a weak inverse relationship was noted; that is, heavier toddlers had lower cardiovascular risks as adults.[5] The risk of cardiovascular morbidity in obese children who became obese adults was lower than in normal-weight children who became obese adults. The authors stated that BMI is a measure of weight relative to height, not actual adiposity, and in children, fat-free mass makes up a higher proportion of BMI compared with adults. They noted that the correlation between BMI and percentage of body fat is lower in children and adolescents compared with adults. The authors felt the lower association between childhood BMI and adult metabolic risk may reflect long-term consequences of differences in the trajectory of lean mass deposition from early childhood.[6]

As previously noted, the vast majority of studies demonstrate increased levels of all-cause as well as specific mortalities attributed to obesity, and at a population level, obesity is estimated to decrease life expectancy up to 7 years.[7] A recent systematic review among adults reported that an increased mortality (hazard ratio, 1.18) was associated with all grades of obesity combined (BMI > 30), and was especially increased (hazard ratio, 1.29) for those with grades 2 and 3 obesity. This study noted that BMI in the overweight range was associated with a slightly lower risk of all-cause mortality (hazard ratio, 0.94).[8] One recent prospective longitudinal study examined Native American children to determine whether BMI, glucose tolerance, blood pressure, and cholesterol levels predicted premature death (before age 55 years). In the mean follow-up period of almost 24 years, death rates from endogenous causes among adults who had been in the highest BMI quartile as children were double those of children in the lowest BMI quartile (incidence-rate ratio, 1.73; 95% confidence interval, 1.09 to 2.74). Obesity, glucose intolerance, and hypertension were strongly associated with increased rates of premature death from endogenous causes, whereas hypercholesterolemia was not a major predictor of this outcome.[9]

Conclusion

Evidence exists that obese children are at increased risk to become obese adults, without an intervention to stop weight gain. We know that obesity predisposes our patients to type 2 diabetes, metabolic syndrome, and PCOS. Obese adults are prone to cardiovascular disease, stroke, and cancers, and obesity may decrease life expectancy by 7 years. Longitudinal studies have shown that obese children had higher premature death rates that were associated with obesity, hypertension, and glucose intolerance. However, the nature of the relationship between childhood obesity (as measured by BMI) and adult disease risk is complex. Those patients who are closer to a normal BMI in childhood but become obese in adulthood appear to be at increased risk. Cardiovascular risk seems to be related more to fitness than body mass, and obese adults who had been obese children may have a lower risk compared with those who became obese in adulthood. Risk of metabolic syndrome may be decreased in obese adults who were obese children due to lean body mass deposition. As care providers for children, we should note current BMI and review these data with families, recommend dietary practices that minimize sweetened beverages and screen time, encourage regular physical activity, and, if the patient is obese, recommend weight loss, or, if that is not possible, weight stabilization.

References

1. Maffeis C, Banzato C, Talamini G. Waist-to-height ratio, a useful index to identify high metabolic risk in overweight children. *J Pediatr.* 2008;152(2):207-213.
2. Bayer O, Krüger H, von Kries R, Toschke AM. Factors associated with tracking of BMI: a meta-regression analysis on BMI tracking. *Obesity (Silver Spring).* 2011;19(5):1069-1076.
3. Singh AS, Mulder C, Twisk JW, van Mechelen W, Chinapaw MJ. Tracking of childhood overweight into adulthood: a systematic review of the literature. *Obes Rev.* 2008;9(5):474-488.
4. Bugge A, El-Naaman B, McMurray RG, Froberg K, Andersen LB. Tracking of clustered cardiovascular disease risk factors from childhood to adolescence. *Pediatr Res.* 2013;73(2)245-249.
5. Owen CG, Whincup PH, Orfei L, et al. Is body mass index before middle age related to coronary heart disease risk in later life? Evidence from observational studies. *Int J Obes (Lond).* 2009;33(8):866-877.
6. Lloyd LJ, Langley-Evans SC, McMullen S. Childhood obesity and risk of the adult metabolic syndrome: a systematic review. *Int J Obes (Lond).* 2012;36(1):1-11.
7. Muennig P, Lubetkin E, Jia H, Franks P. Gender and the burden of disease attributable to obesity. *Am J Public Health.* 2006;96(9):1662-1668.
8. Flegal KM, Kit BK, Orpana H, Graubard BI. Association of all-cause mortality with overweight and obesity using standard body mass index categories: a systematic review and meta-analysis. *JAMA.* 2013;309(1):71-82.
9. Franks PW, Hanson RL, Knowler WC, Sievers ML, Bennett PH, Looker HC. Childhood obesity, other cardiovascular risk factors, and premature death. *N Engl J Med.* 2010;362(6):485-493.

SECTION VI

TREATMENT

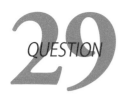

29

WHAT ARE SOME BEHAVIORAL PROGRAMS AVAILABLE FOR OBESE CHILDREN, AND HOW DO I CHOOSE WHICH WOULD BE THE MOST APPROPRIATE FOR MY OBESE PATIENTS?

H. Mollie Grow, MD, MPH

Background

Behavioral programs refer to the cornerstone of obesity treatment: behavior change to adopt healthier lifestyles, including healthy eating, increased physical activity, and decreased sedentary time. This is certainly not an easy task! Most people need external support and structure to make lifestyle changes. (Thus, the appeal of TV shows like *The Biggest Loser*.) Although people continue to seek the elusive magic pill that can make weight loss fast and easy, the reality is that consistent healthy eating and activity habits show the best results for successful weight loss. Although most adults find it quite difficult to lose weight and maintain it, some evidence exists that targeting earlier behavior changes in children may produce better long-term results. In part, this may stem from the fact that before puberty, children are still growing in height and thus even weight maintenance (rather than losing weight) can help improve their body mass index (BMI).[1] Nevertheless, I like to make sure families understand the hopefulness for success by addressing the problem early.

The biggest challenge in many locations remains the availability of obesity treatment programs for youth. Most high-quality programs have been developed through research at universities and/or children's hospitals, thus accessibility is often better in bigger cities. Even where programs are accessible, scheduling availability is often limited, which stems more from funding constraints rather than need. Hopefully, with increased recognition of the benefits from intervening early with obesity, reimbursement for obesity services will improve and more consistent options will be available. In the meantime, being aware of resources in your area can help you address the needs of the approximately 1 in 3 patients you see who are overweight or obese.

Huang JS, ed. *Curbside Consultation in Pediatric Obesity: 49 Clinical Questions* (pp 133-136).
© 2014 Taylor & Francis Group

I have found that it often takes families months to years to accept and then work up the interest (and courage) to get help with their child's weight. Like with smoking cessation, people are in different stages of readiness to address obesity. Frequent check-ins can help families along the stages of change (ie, precontemplation, contemplation, taking action, and maintenance).[1] Although ideally this can be performed at well-child visits, often families who are not ready and/or do not see the importance of change do not show up for or even schedule such appointments, so it can help to discuss weight-related issues even during acute-care visits. In truth, most families will need external help and support of some kind to adopt the lifestyle changes necessary for effective weight management, especially when the child's BMI is already above the 95th percentile and/or when a strong family history of obesity exists.

Types of Programs

Several types of behavioral programs have been evaluated and found promising for overweight and obese children. Although no one program has been identified as the ideal treatment for obese children, several factors have emerged as central elements to high-quality programs to treat obesity. Just like helping families make decisions about choosing an appropriate child care setting, we need to understand the range of program factors and settings to guide patients in obesity treatment.

Currently, the most widely available form of behavioral programs exists within multidisciplinary obesity treatment clinics at children's hospitals or university hospitals across the country. Most of these clinics include physicians, dietitians, exercise specialists, and psychologists and/or social workers. They offer patients broad-based assessments and then typically meet with patients (and their parents) weekly to monthly for 6 months to 1 year (or longer) to set goals and track behavior change and weight status. An example of such a program is the Optimal Weight for Life clinic affiliated with Harvard and Boston Children's Hospital. Published outcomes data are not available for all sites, but several clinics have published promising results and continue to study how best to offer these programs.

The most widely studied and most successful behavioral treatments to date are family-based behavioral treatment programs[2] offered primarily by health psychologists, often through research protocols. These programs use a structured format incorporating behavioral principles based on psychologist Albert Bandura's Social Cognitive Theory. Many clinical programs also offer a group-based form of this treatment in conjunction with clinic visits. These programs typically meet weekly for 3 to 6 months or longer. The principles of treatment include self-monitoring (writing down foods, activity, and weight), environmental control (changing the home environment for foods and activities), and contingency management (using rewards to change behaviors). One dietary approach adopted in many of these programs is a "stoplight" diet—designating "red foods" that most contribute to weight problems and should be eaten only occasionally, "yellow" foods that can be eaten in moderation, and "green" foods (fruits, vegetables, low-fat dairy, and whole grains) that are encouraged as the main proportion of the diet. Some dietitians have objected to labeling foods as good or bad, but I think this approach can be practical and straightforward, and has helped a lot of families learn better eating habits. In terms of weight loss, comprehensive behavioral interventions of medium-to-high intensity (25 or more hours in 6 months) have been shown the most effective with 1.9 to 3.3 kg/m² reductions in BMI for intervention groups as compared with controls at 12 months.[2]

Finally, additional programs are available in community settings that try to incorporate elements of these clinical or research programs. Several have been studied and shown to be successful in reducing BMI. An example is the Bright Bodies program developed at Yale and

---

Table 29-1
Factors in High-Quality Youth Obesity Treatment Programs

- Family-based: Involve parents and focus on changes for the whole family
- Provide moderate- to high-intensity interventions (>25 hours in 6 months are more successful)
- Comprehensive: Include healthy diet counseling, physical activity, and behavioral management techniques (self-monitoring, changing environment)
- Focus on long-term behavioral health changes (sustainable change)
- Use a stepped-care approach: Provide more intensive intervention as weight increases (including considering medications for overweight adolescents)

---

offered at local schools, based on a 12-week healthy eating and activity curriculum called Smart Moves.[3] The curriculum is now being used in a number of other cities in the United States (see http://www.smartmovesforkids.com). Another similar program developed in England called MEND meets twice weekly for 9 weeks and is now being offered in some US cities through YMCAs. It has also shown benefits for BMI reduction.[4] One challenge for most programs is sustainability: when grant funding is finished, the program is no longer available. In my area, I work with a locally developed program called ACT! Actively Changing Together, a 12-week program (similar to the others mentioned) offered in partnership with the YMCA. The program has been available for more than 10 years by sustaining it through training YMCA staff and using YMCA funding and programming infrastructure.

Selection Criteria

You should feel fortunate if choices exist in your area for youth obesity treatment programs. When choices exist, it is important to review what is available with families and provide encouragement and support to try a program. There are a few things to keep in mind when you have options. First, what is the quality of the program? High-quality programs, as described by the US Preventive Services Task Force, include several factors (Table 29-1). If a comprehensive, high-quality treatment program is not available in your area, refer to a structured exercise/physical activity program for an activity the child likes to do. No matter what weight a patient is, physical activity provides multiple benefits, including improved mood and sleep and prevention of weight-related comorbidities like hypertension and diabetes.

Another factor is the feasibility of programs for your patients' families. Low-income families need accessible programs that are designed to work for them; I suggest some criteria to consider in Table 29-2. Most programs have been tested in more affluent and educated populations. Additional research is needed to determine which programs best support diverse families. When available, community-based programs are ideal because they are often tailored to engage families close to where they live.

Table 29-2

Suggested Criteria for Obesity Treatment Programs Serving Diverse, Low-Income Families

- Close to home
- Free or low cost (sliding-scale fees)
- Provide activities for the whole family
- Child care available for younger children
- Accommodate schedules of working parents
- Flexible times for enrollment/participation
- Materials available in multiple languages

On the Horizon

Many areas still have little available for youth obesity treatment. For families in rural areas, traveling to a big city for weekly treatment is not feasible. One more recent approach by some programs has been adopting mobile technologies to reach families. For example, some clinics have telehealth options for pediatric obesity, such as UC Davis' Healthy Eating-Active Living Telehealth program. Other programs are incorporating text messaging and smartphones that have apps for weight reduction. Hopefully, more creative options like this will soon be available to all of our families at costs that are feasible regardless of socioeconomic status.

References

1. Barlow SE; Expert Committee. Expert committee recommendations regarding the prevention, assessment, and treatment of child and adolescent overweight and obesity: summary report. *Pediatrics*. 2007;120(Suppl 4): S164-S192.
2. Whitlock EP, O'Connor EA, Williams SB, Beil TL, Lutz KW. Effectiveness of weight management interventions in children: a targeted systematic review for the USPSTF. *Pediatrics*. 2010;125(2):e396-e418.
3. Savoye M, Nowicka P, Shaw M, et al. Long-term results of an obesity program in an ethnically diverse pediatric population. *Pediatrics*. 2011;127(3):402-410.
4. Sacher PM, Kolotourou M, Chadwick PM, et al. Randomized controlled trial of the MEND program: a family-based community intervention for childhood obesity. *Obesity (Silver Spring)*. 2010;18(Suppl 1):S62-S68.

30
QUESTION

THERE ARE MANY DIETS OUT THERE TO "TREAT" OBESITY. WHICH ONE(S) SHOULD I RECOMMEND? WHICH HAVE DEMONSTRATED EFFECTIVENESS?

Karen Stephens, MS, RD, CSP, LD and Sarah Hampl, MD

With the continual stream of media reports touting magical solutions for weight loss or announcements of breakthroughs, you may wonder why more of your patients are obese and what the solution is. It would be easy to hand a family a diet sheet, wish them good luck, and hope for the best. However, obesity is a complex condition with cultural, emotional, and social contributors that need to be taken into consideration. Plans for any dietary modifications need to be uncomplicated and realistic for the entire family. We want families to learn to use real foods to build a healthy diet. Our favorite plans are those using a balance of macronutrients such as MyPlate,[1] the traffic light diet, a reduced glycemic load diet, and, occasionally, a low-carbohydrate diet.

We prefer the balanced macronutrient diets because they provide a variety of nutrients from all food groups; include carbohydrate, protein, and fat; and establish a foundation for long-term healthy lifestyle change. Our favorite is the plate model, which was first used as a means of teaching healthy eating to people with diabetes. A family is taught to divide a 9-inch plate into 4 sections and place the correct food group in each compartment, not stacked higher than 1 inch. We counsel patients to fill half the plate with nonstarchy vegetables such as lettuce, cucumbers, broccoli, cauliflower, green beans, carrots, spinach, and cabbage; one-fourth of the plate with high-protein foods such as lean poultry or meat, low-fat cheese, beans, eggs, or nuts; and the remaining one-fourth with whole wheat bread or starch such as pasta, rice, potatoes, corn, lima beans, or peas. One cup of skim or 1% milk plus a small serving of fruit is included on the side.

Numerous variations of the balanced macronutrient diet exist, including MyPlate[1] (Figure 30-1) and the Idaho Plate Method, but all are built on the concept of eating foods from all food groups in moderate portions. MyPlate recommends half a plate of vegetables and fruits instead of half a plate of vegetables. This may be more realistic for some families who seldom eat any of one food group or the other.

Huang JS, ed. *Curbside Consultation in Pediatric Obesity: 49 Clinical Questions* (pp 137-140).
© 2014 Taylor & Francis Group

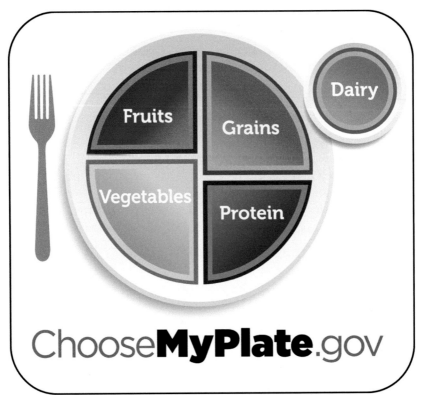

Figure 30-1. MyPlate is one simple plate model for choosing foods from each food group in controlled portions. (Reprinted from the US Department of Agriculture.)

Positives of the plate model are that it provides a sufficient volume of food to promote satiety as well as a variety of food groups to prevent boredom and diet burnout. Eating fruits, vegetables, and whole grains provides dietary fiber, which is filling and improves bowel health. With an emphasis on choices more than on calories or points, families do not have to adopt a diet mentality or engage in all-or-nothing eating. There is automatic portion control if used correctly, unless large second servings are included. Calories are reduced unless individuals choose high-fat and high-sugar choices. Some families use divided plates, which help them remember to choose from all food groups. A real bonus is that young children can learn and apply this visual method of making healthy food choices. They enjoy learning about the food group compartments and are able to fill in the blanks—just like a puzzle.

The traffic light or stoplight diet, developed by Leonard Epstein and colleagues, is another example of a balanced micronutrient diet. It includes foods that are divided into 5 categories: protein; milk and dairy products; grains, including breads, cereal, and starches; fruits and vegetables; and fats and sweets. Each category is assigned a color. The traffic light icon is something that children and parents can easily recognize and understand—green means go, yellow means slow down, and red means stop. When foods are classified as green, yellow, and red, families have a visual image in their minds and learn that green foods are low in calories but high in nutrients, yellow foods are higher in calories but also have plenty of nutrients, and red foods are high in sugar and fat with few other nutrients. Generally, families are encouraged to eat as desired from the green foods, have a set amount of yellow foods, and limit red foods to approximately 4 per week. The goal is to get the most nutrients with the least calories.

The key to weight loss using the traffic light diet is restricted calories, usually in the range of 900 to 1500 calories per day for children. Participants are encouraged to remove all red foods from their homes and to eat mainly green and yellow foods. Families need instructional materials that explicitly list foods, grouped by color for easy reference, with a programmed prescription of choices to stay within the set calories provided and to limit red foods to less than 4 per week. The traffic light diet was part of Epstein's family intervention programs that included self-monitoring, family modeling, praise, involvement of a therapist, and contracting and monetary rewards. Epstein's groups demonstrated modest weight loss over 5 to 10 years, and it is difficult to ascertain the true effects of the diet compared with the other parts of the intervention.[2] The traffic light concept was also used in the 2005 National Institutes of Health childhood obesity and prevention program We Can, with a Go, Slow, Whoa food list based on green, yellow, and red foods.[3] Families are able to graphically see red, yellow, and green choices side by side. It is fun to watch families have "aha" moments when they see how they can change their red food choices to yellow and hopefully to green. For example, simply switching fruits canned in heavy syrup to foods canned in light syrup to fresh or frozen fruits makes the transition from red to green.

Another diet plan that works well for some families is the low glycemic diet. This diet is based on choosing foods with a low glycemic index (GI). The GI is a list that ranks foods from 0 to 100 depending on how quickly they raise blood glucose. The diet is based on choosing foods with a low GI (high-fiber, least-processed grains, fruit, vegetables, and legumes) along with lean meats and healthy fats. There is no counting calories, fats, or carbohydrates. Proponents believe that satiety is increased and blood glucose levels are more stable, avoiding cycling up and down of glucose and insulin levels. It is likely that the main effect on weight is from decreased energy intake as a result of limiting high-sugar foods. One way to teach the low glycemic diet is to use the stoplight icon with low, moderate, and high GI foods to help families make healthy choices. Choosing high-fiber foods and foods in their most natural state as well as avoiding sugar-sweetened drinks will promote high-nutrient, low energy-dense eating.

The GI has limitations because GI lists do not contain all foods and also give the impression that a food has a single value. The GI varies depending on the ripeness of a fruit or how a vegetable is prepared and is influenced by other foods a person eats at the same time. But does that really matter if it helps people choose whole grains, fruits, and vegetables instead of candy, cookies, and chips? Some families may adopt an anti-carb attitude, believing that carbohydrate-containing foods such as potatoes and bread are bad. Carbohydrates are an important part of a healthy diet, and learning to avoid the poor-quality carbs is an important key to healthy choices. Families' ability to maintain a low GI diet over the long term is unknown, but a 2007 Cochrane Review reported that patients eating an ad lib low GI diet in the short term lost more weight and had more improvement in blood lipids than those eating a conventional low-fat decreased-energy diet.[4]

The very low-carbohydrate diet (VLCD) contains 20 to 60 g carbohydrates per day and is sometimes used for short term weight loss treatment for adolescents. The diet includes mainly meats, eggs, cheese, oils, and nonstarchy vegetables in the induction phase, then gradually adds in nuts, berries, legumes, more fruits, starchy vegetables, and limited whole-grain products over several weeks. The VLCD is based on the goal of creating ketosis by restricting carbohydrate intake and subsequently using fat as the body's energy source instead of stored glycogen. Monitoring urine for ketones is one method of ensuring compliance with the diet. Working closely with a registered dietitian is also important if prescribing a VLCD.

Typically with low carbohydrate intake, an initial water loss shows up as rapid weight loss. This may provide motivation for teens to continue the diet. Another benefit of eating foods high in protein and fat is the longer digestion time that decreases appetite and increases feelings of fullness. This may help cut down on mindless eating that provides excess calories. Also, by restricting foods containing high levels of carbohydrate, energy-dense foods such as cookies, pastries, candy, chips, crackers, and bread are eliminated, leading to reduced calorie consumption. A 2012 study at Boston Children's Hospital compared the Atkins Diet (VLCD), a low GI diet, and a low-fat, high-carbohydrate diets. Results reported the least reduction in resting metabolic rate and the highest total energy expenditure with the VLCD. The negative results with the VLCD were higher levels of C-reactive protein, which may be a marker for future cardiovascular disease.[5] However, controversy remains regarding the VLCD and its effects on long-term health. A stricter VLCD is the protein-sparing modified fast for rapid weight loss in morbidly obese individuals. The protein-sparing modified fast diet is a hypocaloric diet (600 to 800 kcal/day), which severely restricts carbohydrates and includes 1.5 to 2 gm/kg ideal body weight of high-quality protein up to 100 grams per day, including lean meats, seafood, egg whites, and poultry. Effectiveness has been shown in children,[6] but diet performance must be monitored closely by an experienced dietitian under medical supervision and is limited in duration. Fluids, vitamins, and mineral supplements must be provided to prevent dehydration and nutrient deficiency.

Dietary habits are difficult to change because eating represents family traditions, cultures, and ways of expressing love and other emotions. No matter what the approach, nothing works well without parental support and family changes in eating and activity habits. Children of obese parents have an approximately 80% chance of also being obese.[7] Without parents making an effort to improve their own health habits, children will not succeed. The basic health habits of eating breakfast, avoiding sugar-sweetened drinks, increasing vegetables and fruits, and eating meals and controlled snacks provide a foundation for more specific dietary changes. Then, as a family tries a balanced plate method or a low glycemic program, they will make positive strides.

References

1. US Department of Agriculture. ChooseMyPlate.gov. http://www.choosemyplate.gov/print-materials-ordering/graphic-resources.html. Accessed January 10, 2013.
2. Academy of Nutrition and Dietetics Evidence Analysis Library. The Traffic Light Diet and Treating Childhood Obesity. http://andevidencelibrary.com/evidence.cfm?evidence_summary_id=250033&auth=1. Accessed January 7, 2013.
3. US Department of Health and Human Services, National Institutes of Health, National Heart, Lung, and Blood Institute. We Can! GO, SLOW, and WHOA Foods. http://www.nhlbi.nih.gov/health/public/heart/obesity/wecan/eat-right/choosing-foods.htm. Accessed January 10, 2013.
4. Thomas DE, Elliott EJ, Baur L. Low glycaemic index or low glycaemic load diets for overweight and obesity. *Cochrane Database Syst Rev.* 2007;3:CD005105.
5. Ebbeling C, Swain JF, Feldman HA, et al. Effects of dietary composition on energy expenditure during weight-loss maintenance. *JAMA.* 2012;307(24):2627-2634.
6. Suskind RM, Blecker U, Udall JN Jr, et al. Recent advances in the treatment of childhood obesity. *Pediatr Diabetes.* 2000;1:23-33.
7. Whitaker RC, Wright JA, Pepe MS, Seidel KD, Dietz WH. Predicting obesity in young adulthood from childhood and parental obesity. *N Engl J Med.* 1997;337:869–873.

My Patients Often Ask Me About Fad Diets for Weight Loss. What Is the Bottom Line About Fad Diets? Are They Benign, or Do Some Have Associated Adverse Risks?

Rohit Gupta, MD, PhD and David L. Suskind, MD

Fad diets sound great, and they would be great if they worked, but fad diets don't work, and certainly not for long-term weight loss. In truth, most people quickly regain the lost weight, sometimes adding even more pounds to their baseline weight. In addition, although fad diets are often benign, some carry the risks of serious complications, which cannot be overlooked.

Etiology

Fad diets are the result of a major unfulfilled need in the United States and other industrialized countries, combined with an eye toward making a profit. The steady rise in the average body mass index across all age groups coupled with recognition of associated health consequences in the last few decades has spurred a need to trim down, both for health and esthetic reasons. This need has given rise to a massive market for diets that are "fast" and "really work." Although this chapter cannot describe every one of the hundreds of fad diets on the market, their common strategies can be analyzed. Almost universally, marketplace fad diets rely on unusual combinations of foods and/or eating patterns often combined with novel additions that, theoretically, directly cause weight reduction. All fad diets claim immediate or rapid weight loss. They are, according to their commercials and infomercials, "effective for all." They attract not only the obese and overweight but also individuals who would simply like to lose a few pounds. The economic impact has been enormous, while the results have been far less satisfying.

Huang JS, ed. *Curbside Consultation in Pediatric Obesity: 49 Clinical Questions* (pp 141-143).
© 2014 Taylor & Francis Group

Fad Diets

The basic premise for weight loss in fad diets is extreme caloric restriction. Fad diets typically have a caloric content ranging from 200 kcal per day to 800 kcal per day. Their various methods often gain publicity by word of mouth, bulletin boards, Web-based advertising, or unsolicited e-mailing. The grapefruit diet, for example, which uses either the whole fruit or the juice, has been around since the 1930s. Repopularized in the 1980s as the 10 day-10 pound weight reduction diet, the diet touted effectiveness via the faulty assumption that grapefruits both decreased insulin levels and had fat-burning enzymes. Ultimately, this was proven untrue, with the demonstrated short-term weight loss effectiveness of eating grapefruit before meals eventually attributed to a low energy-dense dietary preload. In the scientific domain, however, there has been some interest in studying the effect of grapefruit on weight loss. Two known compounds, naringenin and nootkatone, found in higher concentrations in grapefruit, are currently being studied as mediators of grapefruit's potential effects on weight loss. That potential notwithstanding, it is important to remember that grapefruit has significant interactions with medications such as statins, anti-arrhythmics, immunosuppressants, and antihypertensives (calcium channel blockers), with the known potential of fatal complications.[1]

The lemonade diet, also known as the master cleanse diet, claims to detoxify the body and remove excess fat. Patients are restricted to consuming only liquids made from a mixture of tea, lemonade, maple syrup, and cayenne pepper. Significantly deficient in proteins, vitamins, and minerals, the lemonade diet has the potential of wreaking havoc on the dieter's health, especially for children, teens, and pregnant or breastfeeding women. Most individuals will suffer from significant diarrhea, dizziness, and nausea. In addition, after stopping the diet, regaining the weight back is almost ensured.

The relatively newer chocolate diet embraces the idea of consuming as much chocolate as the individual desires with the underlying premise to lose weight, presumably a direct effect of chocolate intake. This diet has gained popularity based on the idea that chocolate contains compounds that aid in burning calories, with the added benefit of antioxidants. Although chocolate is made from processing cacao beans that are rich in monounsaturated fats and flavonoids as antioxidants, the chocolate diet works only when total calories are restricted to less than 800 kcal. This raises the question of whether it is the chocolate or the calorie restriction.

Fruitarianism is a diet dependent on eliminating all animal products and vegetables and consuming only fruits, nuts, and seeds. Fruitarianism has not been shown to result in weight loss. What it has been shown to produce are serious deficiencies in protein, essential fatty acids, vitamins B12 and D, and minerals such as calcium and zinc.

Efficacy

Fad diets (ie, very low-calorie diets), when compared with conventional diets, have been shown to result in short-term weight loss. This is attributable to their extreme caloric restrictions; no particular component, whether herbs, fruits, chemicals, etc, has ever been shown to be responsible for the weight loss. In the short term, individuals who adhered to very low-calorie diets have demonstrated reduction in blood pressures and marked improvement in hyperglycemia. However, in the long term, weight loss was not maintained, and individuals often regained and increased their overall weight.

Side Effects

Almost always, fad diets are self-administered, with little or no medical supervision. The potential health risks cannot be dismissed easily. For all fad dieters, there is the problem of decreased energy, a sensation of cold due to loss of adipose tissue insulation, hair loss due to decreased protein intake, skin thinning, and loss of muscle mass. For individuals on antihypertensive medications, very low-calorie diets can result in a drastic fall in blood pressure and symptomatic hypotension episodes, mostly during the first week. For diabetics, the long-term effects of severe caloric restriction include mobilization of cholesterol from fat stores, which may result in increased gallstone formation, necessitating surgical intervention. In addition, increased glucose monitoring is essential for diabetics who are restricting their carbohydrate (glucose) intake because it can potentially lead to clinically significant episodes of hypoglycemia. Because of negative effects on the developing fetus or the newborn, very low-calorie fad diets are absolutely contraindicated in pregnant or nursing women. Similarly, very low-calorie diets are contraindicated in children and teenagers because their linear and developmental growth depends on protein and other nutrient intake that is lacking in most fad diets.[2]

The need to lose weight fast is a psychological one. For those who are obese or even somewhat overweight, the promoted goal should be the achievement of a healthy weight and its long-term maintenance. This requires a diet that provides appropriate calories for healthy weight loss, allows achievement of a healthy weight goal, and enables a recipe for lifetime maintenance. The real long-term goal is, after all, to be healthy, both in appearance and organically. An unproven fad diet may look good in the ads and even produce short-term weight loss but may prove to be harmful or ineffective in the long term. The role of the professional is to understand the need to lose weight fast, present a dietary plan that makes sense to the individual and his or her lifestyle, and offer the supervision and support to help make the plan work.

References

1. Pirmohamed M. Drug-grapefruit juice interactions: two mechanisms are clear but individual responses vary. *BMJ*. 2013;346:f1.
2. Tsai AG, Wadden TA. The evolution of very-low-calorie diets: an update and meta-analysis. *Obesity (Silver Spring)*. 2006;14(8):1283-1293.

HOW CAN A PRIMARY CARE PRACTITIONER MANAGE OBESITY? WHAT SPECIALISTS ARE AVAILABLE TO HELP, AND WHEN SHOULD REFERRAL BE CONSIDERED?

Sandra Hassink, MD, FAAP

Primary care practitioners are in the ideal position to help families and children prevent and treat childhood obesity. The primary care encounter is one of the few places that families and children have the opportunity to address healthy nutrition and activity behaviors together, address the health impact of obesity, and work to create family-centered solutions with the expert partnership of their primary care provider. The advantages of addressing obesity in primary care are the early and continuous relationship that the practitioner establishes with the child and family, the knowledge the primary care clinician has of the child's environment, and the ability of the provider to guide family-based change over time. To accomplish this, the provider must be willing to incorporate obesity management into office training and workflow.

The Expert Committee[1] recommendations provide a framework for addressing the continuum of childhood obesity, from primary prevention to tertiary care. In primary care, the steps the clinician needs to take to incorporate obesity management into the office routine are (1) establish the routines necessary to calculate, chart, and classify body mass index (BMI) for all children aged 2 to 18 years and weight for height for children aged 0 to 2 years, at least yearly; (2) understand the major prevention and treatment strategies that can be used to achieve a healthy weight; (3) be able to assess child and family dietary patterns and nutritional environment both at well-child and follow-up visits; (4) incorporate the assessment of physical activity and sedentary behavior into routine screening; (5) evaluate the readiness of the families to change and assess their need for information and skills; (6) identify the presence and extent of obesity-related comorbidities and have a plan to address them; and (7) have the ability to assess ongoing progress.

Huang JS, ed. *Curbside Consultation in
Pediatric Obesity: 49 Clinical Questions* (pp 145-150).
© 2014 Taylor & Francis Group

The calculation of BMI (kg/m2) is a screening measure that can help clinicians determine the need for further evaluation. The BMI is based on age and sex and is a population-based reference. Current recommendations are to use the 2000 Centers for Disease Control growth charts for children aged 2 to 20 years and the World Health Organization growth charts for children aged 0 to 2 years.[2] BMI is classified according to percentiles, with BMI < 5% classified as underweight; BMI 5% to 84% as normal weight; BMI 85% to 94% as overweight; and BMI ≥ 95% as obesity. Growth charts should be reviewed with families in detail because they may not know how to interpret them.[3] The introduction to the growth chart can be an opportunity to introduce the topic of unhealthy weight/obesity and increase families' familiarity and comfort with routinely discussing these measures.

Understanding major prevention and treatment strategies to achieve a healthy weight is an important foundation for performing a dietary and activity assessment. Multiple studies show consistent association between the following recommended behaviors and either obesity risk or energy balance: limited or no consumption of sugar-sweetened beverages, limiting TV viewing (0 hours for children younger than 2 years, < 2 hours for children older than 2 years), removing the TV from the primary sleeping area, eating breakfast daily, limiting eating out, eating family meals, eating appropriate portion sizes, getting adequate sleep, and breastfeeding.

The following are additional health behaviors that could support healthy weight: eating a diet rich in calcium; eating a diet high in fiber, eating a diet with balanced macronutrients (food groups), engaging in moderate-vigorous activity 60 minutes/day, and limiting consumption of energy-dense foods. These strategies are recommended by the Expert Committee as prevention and treatment strategies.

Taking advantage of well-child visits to initiate discussions about healthy lifestyle is one of the key strategies for intervening in the obesity epidemic. The Expert Committee considered all children at risk for obesity and encouraged focus on reduction of high-risk behaviors. Messages should be simple and consistent and should take advantage of the clinician's ability to institute cumulative prevention strategies over time.

Many clinicians have found that adopting a message such as 5210, which stands for at least 5 fruit and vegetable servings/day, no more than 2 hours of recreational screen time, 1 hour of physical activity, and 0 sugar drinks, is a convenient way to start the conversation about high-risk behaviors, provides actionable targets for change, and can be an entry point for other important behavior change strategies.

It is important to recognize that family-centered care is at the core of childhood obesity treatment. Encouraging the entire family to set goals for and adopt healthy lifestyle behaviors is essential to supporting the child. Family-based strategies such as keeping a healthy kitchen, eating family meals, establishing eating and sleeping routines, and supporting positive and effective parenting are all important in sustaining change.

Comorbidities of obesity are common and often require involvement of multidisciplinary providers and pediatric subspecialists. Table 32-1 lists common comorbidities, symptoms, and pertinent subspecialty involvement.

Obesity-related emergencies, although rare, are increasingly being seen and primary care practitioners and office staff should be alert to their presentations. A few specific emergency situations are described next.

Hyperglycemic Hyperosmolar Syndrome

Patients with unrecognized type 2 diabetes mellitus (a common comorbidity with obesity) can present with hyperglycemic hyperosmolar syndrome and can have symptoms preceding metabolic decompensation of vomiting, abdominal pain, dizziness, weakness, polyuria, polydipsia, weight loss, and diarrhea. Practitioners should be alert and respond to these complaints in patients with obesity. American Diabetes Association criteria for hyperglycemic hyperosmolar syndrome include serum glucose concentration > 600 mg/dL, arterial pH > 7.3, serum bicarbonate > 19 mEq/L, small urine and serum ketones, effective serum osmolality > 320 mOsm/kg, variable anion gap, and neurologic abnormalities including coma.

Diabetic Ketoacidosis

Diabetic ketoacidosis can also be a presentation of type 2 diabetes mellitus. If basal insulin secretion is low, there is increasing susceptibility to relative insulin deficiency. Insulin resistance combined with chronic hyperglycemia and decreasing insulin secretion results in relative insulin deficiency. When deficiency becomes severe, this leads to enhanced lipolysis and increased levels of free fatty acids, ketonemia, and ketonuria.

Pulmonary Embolism

Pulmonary embolism has been reported in adolescents with obesity. Risk factors include obesity hypoventilation syndrome, coagulation disorder, and bariatric surgery.

Bariatric Surgery

Bariatric surgery is becoming more common in the adolescent population. Practitioners need to be alert for both early (postsurgical, obstructive) and late (nutritional, obstructive) postoperative complications. Generally, monitoring is performed in conjunction with the surgical team and/or with a pediatric gastroenterologist.

Table 32-1

Common Comorbidities, Symptoms, and Pertinent Subspecialty Involvement

Comorbidity	Symptoms	Signs	Evaluation and Treatment	Subspecialty
Pseudotumor cerebri (idiopathic intracranial hypertension) *Requires emergency treatment*	Headache, visual impairment, vomiting, neck, shoulder, back pain	Papilledema, visual impairment	Rule out other causes of increased intracranial pressure Acetazolamide, lumboperitoneal shunt Weight loss	Neurology Ophthalmology Neurosurgery
Obstructive sleep apnea	Snoring, daytime tiredness, poor school performance, napping, nighttime awakening, enuresis	Snoring, restless sleep, nighttime apnea	Nighttime polysomnography CPaP or BiPAP Weight loss	Ear, nose, throat Pulmonology
NASH	Asymptomatic or mild right upper quadrant discomfort	Elevated AST/ALT	Exclude other causes of liver disease Liver biopsy Weight loss	Hepatology Gastroenterology
Cholelithiasis	Abdominal pain, nausea, tenderness	Right upper quadrant tenderness, elevated liver function studies	Exclude other causes of abdominal pain Abdominal ultrasound	Gastroenterology Pediatric surgeon
Polycystic ovarian syndrome	Oligomenorrhea or amenorrhea, hirsutism, acne, history of premature adrenarche	Hirsutism, acne, elevated androgens insulin resistance, glucose intolerance, type 2 diabetes	Evaluate for metabolic syndrome and diabetes Weight loss Metformin Oral contraceptives	Adolescent medicine Endocrinology
Type 2 diabetes	Polyuria; polydipsia; nocturia; recurrent vaginal, bladder, or other infections; recent weight loss	*Acanthosis nigricans*	Fasting glucose ≥126 mg/dlL, 2 hour plasma glucose ≥200 mg/dL (OGTT), random plasma glucose ≥200 mg/dL, hemoglobin A1c ≥6.5% Exclude type 1 diabetes Metformin; insulin; weight loss	Endocrinology

(continued)

Table 32-1 (continued)

Common Comorbidities, Symptoms, and Pertinent Subspecialty Involvement

Comorbidity	Symptoms	Signs	Evaluation and Treatment	Subspecialty
Dyslipidemia	Asymptomatic, associated with other obesity-related comorbidities	Acanthosis nigricans	Elevated cholesterol and/or elevated triglycerides, low HDL cholesterol Dietary management Pharmacologic management	Cardiology
Hypertension	Asymptomatic	Elevated systolic or diastolic blood pressure	Exclude other causes of hypertension Evaluate for other obesity-related comorbidities Recommend diet high in fruits and vegetables, low salt, weight loss	Cardiology Nephrology
Slipped capital femoral epiphysis *Requires emergency treatment*	Hip or knee pain Limp	Pain on hip or knee examination Limp	Bilateral hip radiographs Immediate surgery	Orthopedics
Blount disease	Bowing, knee pain, limp	Bowing, pain on knee examination, limp	Knee radiographs Surgery	Orthopedics
Depression	Family history of depression, psychological trauma, teasing/bullying, low self-esteem	Loss of interest, anger, irritability, sadness, suicidal ideation, lack of self-care	Depression screen/evaluation	Psychology Psychiatry

Abbreviations: ALT, alanine aminotransferase; AST, aspartate aminotransferase; BiPAP, bilevel positive airway pressure; CPaP, continuous positive airway pressure; HDL, high-density lipoprotein; NASH, nonalcoholic steatohepatitis; OGTT, oral glucose tolerance test.

References

1. Barlow SE; Expert Committee. Expert committee recommendations regarding the prevention, assessment, and treatment of child and adolescent overweight and obesity: summary report. *Pediatrics*. 2007;120(Suppl 4):S164-S192.
2. Grummer-Strawn LM, Reinold C, Krebs NF. Use of the World Health Organization and CDC growth charts for children aged 0-59 months in the United States. *MMWR Recomm Rep*. 2010;59(RR-9):1-15.
3. Ben-Joseph EP, Dowshen SA, Izenberg N. Do parents understand growth charts? A national, Internet-based survey. *Pediatrics*. 2009;124(4):1100-1109.

WHAT IS MOTIVATIONAL INTERVIEWING, AND HOW CAN I USE IT TO HELP MOTIVATE MY PATIENTS TO LOSE WEIGHT?

Kyung E. Rhee, MD, MSc, MA and Abby L. Braden, PhD

Motivational interviewing (MI) is a style of counseling used to help people who are ambivalent or resistant about making a behavior change. In the clinical setting, it is often termed *behavior change counseling*. Although it was originally used to treat addictions, it has been used with many other chronic diseases and behaviors, such as diabetes management, HIV medication adherence, smoking cessation, increasing dietary adherence, and sunscreen use.[1] This counseling method has been described as a "person-centered method of guiding to elicit and strengthen personal motivation for change."[2(p137)] However, it is different from traditional Rogerian talk therapy in that it is much more goal-oriented with a focus on positive behavioral outcomes. It is this more directed nature of the interaction that allows it to be amenable for use in the clinical setting, where time restrictions are great.

Although MI in the clinical setting is often broken down into strategies or techniques that can be used to assess and draw out patients' ideas about change, an underlying tone exists that should not be forgotten. In successful MI encounters, providers are skilled at empathic listening and avoid judging the patient or proscribing what the patient should do. They use reflective listening skills, open-ended questions, and affirming statements to support patients as they articulate their reasons for or against change. This supportive and collaborative environment surrounding the encounter is essential if patients are to feel comfortable enough to discuss their opinions openly and explore their ambivalence. When providers act as authoritarian figures and insist or scare patients into making changes, patients often feel attacked and subsequently shut down any thought of making a change. Instead, providers will make more headway if they cultivate a feeling of collaboration with patients in such a way that the patients set the pace and direction of the care and interaction. As a result, patients will feel like they have control over the process and that they are supported. They will then do most of the psychological work to ready themselves to make a change and, in the end, will be more likely to reach the point at which change occurs.

Huang JS, ed. *Curbside Consultation in Pediatric Obesity: 49 Clinical Questions* (pp 151-154).
© 2014 Taylor & Francis Group

Table 33-1

Comparison of Encounters That Use Traditional Counseling Methods and Motivational Interviewing

Traditional Encounter	Motivational Interviewing
• Physician acts as the expert	• Patient is expert regarding his or her behaviors
• Physician is responsible for change—directive interaction	• Patient is responsible for change—collaborative interaction
• Physician does most of the talking	• Patient does most of the talking to resolve ambivalence
• Physician labels or confronts (eg, "This is a problem")	• Explore patient's views regarding the behavior
• Premature focus and discussion around change behaviors	• Explore reasons for/against change, develop a discrepancy, support self-efficacy to change
• Warn, preach, persuade, lecture	• Uses empathic counseling style to evoke change
• Provide answers or solutions	• Provides a menu of change options and advice on how to change behaviors

The overall goals for the physician, therefore, are to support patients as they go through this process; try to evoke change rather than educate, preach, or force them to change; and collaborate with the patient. Physicians too often believe it is their responsibility to make people adopt healthier lifestyle behaviors. However, if you remember that the patient is an autonomous person who needs to come to the decision that he or she wants to change on his or her own, then your approach to the session will take on a different tone, one that is less confrontational and preachy and may provide more satisfaction and efficacy in the long run (Table 33-1). Ultimately, in a successful MI encounter, you are primarily there to help support the patient in this change process and provide recommendations only when the patient is ready to change.

Keeping this in mind, when you begin an MI encounter, it is often beneficial to get the patient's permission to discuss the topic of interest and understand how the targeted behavior fits into the patient's current lifestyle. In the case of an overweight child, the parent (we will presume mother for this discussion) is often the agent of change, and it would behoove you to tell the mother that you are concerned with her child's weight and would like to discuss the matter further with her. Once she agrees to this discussion, ask open-ended questions to get a feeling as to whether the mother agrees that the child's weight is of concern and what behaviors she thinks are contributing to this problem. This process will allow you to proceed more appropriately with the subsequent dialogue. If she does not think that her child's weight is an issue, you know then to tailor the conversation around why you think this is an issue and what concerns you have for the child. However, if the mother agrees that the child is overweight but never thought about or knew how to make a change to her diet, a different conversation would ensue. (For the purposes of brevity, "patient" in the subsequent discussion will refer to either or both the child and parent.)

	Pros/Benefits	Cons/Costs
If I don't change	1. 2. 3.	1. 2. 3.
If I do change	1. 2. 3.	1. 2. 3.

Figure 33-1. The pros and cons of making a change using a decisional balance grid.

While maintaining the spirit of collaboration, you can then probe (using open-ended questions and reflective listening techniques) for reasons that personally motivate the patient to change. However, there are often times when patients have few reasons to change or are resistant to change. In that case, you can guide the patient to explore reasons for and against making a behavior change by asking him or her about the pros and cons of making a change and not making a change (Figure 33-1). The patient will hopefully see that the pros of making a change outweigh the pros of not making a change (or the cons of not making a change have a greater consequence than the cons of making a change). This process of decisional balance is designed to enhance intrinsic motivation through the use of change talk, a process by which the patient reflects on the discrepancies between his or her values or views of him- or herself and what the behaviors are actually reflecting of him- or herself. For example, the mother of an overweight or obese child may value her child's health but frequently provide foods high in fat and sugar to the child. This does not reflect the behavior of a parent committed to her child's health. Highlighting this discrepancy between the patient's values and behavior often results in the patient trying to resolve the discrepancy. This discussion can often move a patient toward wanting to make a change, or to at least be willing to think about making a behavior change. In addition to this method, you may want to ask the patient to project into the future and imagine what life would be like if he or she did or did not make a change. For some patients who are able to think in the long term, this exercise may motivate them to make a behavior change.

Two other important questions that are often asked of patients in these sessions are (1) how important is it for you to make this change, and (2) how confident are you that you can make a change (Figure 33-2)? These questions allow you to assess the patient's readiness to make a change. If the mother thinks it is important to make a change but doesn't think she can do it, then you as the provider know to focus on supporting her confidence and efficacy to make a change. On the other hand, many patients are confident that they could make a change if they wanted to but don't think it's important enough to do so. In that case, most of your efforts should be focused on helping patients discover relevant personal reasons for making a change. Moving patients along this readiness-to-change continuum often involves exploring their ambivalence, why it is they don't think it's important to make a change, or why they aren't capable of making a change. For patients who report low levels of importance or confidence, it is important to frame their responses positively and ask them why they reported a 2 rather than a 1. In this manner, you are praising them for having some level of confidence or importance, albeit low. This will help the patient frame his or her level of importance or confidence in a somewhat positive frame and prime him

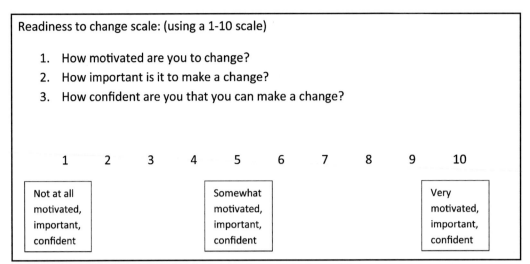

Figure 33-2. Readiness to change scale that can be used during an MI encounter.

or her for your next question of, "What would it take to get you from a 2 to a 3 or 4?" The patient is now pushed to think about what behaviors, thoughts, or feelings would have to change if he or she were to make a change. By not comparing level of readiness with a higher number (like 9 or 10), you also allow the patient to think in smaller, more feasible steps and avoid the possibility of scaring him or her away from the behavior change process. This conversation is just one more step toward highlighting the discrepancy and helping resolve the patient's ambivalence toward change.

So, in the true spirit of MI, the physician does not convince patients to make a change. Instead, the provider should guide patients to think about their own reasons for and against change and how those decisions will affect future goals, current values, or views of themselves. One must also remember that although the ultimate goal is to achieve behavior change, not all patients will reach that stage. Nevertheless, having an open-minded conversation about their views can be enlightening in itself and provide you with more insight and direction for future conversations. When interacting with parents of overweight children, a successful encounter can be one that gets a parent who has never thought about making changes to dietary behaviors to start thinking about the possibility of change. Because MI places the responsibility for change on the patient, and only the patient who is intrinsically motivated can make a change, this process can occur at a much slower pace. However, if the lines of communication are open between provider and patient and this process can continue over time, the patient may someday be ready to make a change. At that point, since the motivation to change was intrinsically generated, the likelihood of successful behavior change will increase. Several references that may be useful are listed next.[3-5]

References

1. Dunn C, Deroo L, Rivara FP. The use of brief interventions adapted from motivational interviewing across behavioral domains: a systematic review. *Addiction.* 2001;96(12):1725-1742.
2. Miller WR, Rollnick S. Ten things that motivational interviewing is not. *Behav Cogn Psychother.* 2009;37(2):129-149.
3. Miller WR, Rollnick S. *Motivational Interviewing: Preparing People for Change.* 2nd ed. New York, NY: The Guilford Press; 2002.
4. Rollnick S, Mason P, Butler C. *Health Behavior Change: A Guide for Practitioners.* 3rd ed. Edinburgh, Scottland: Churchill Livingstone; 2002.
5. Rollnick S. Behavior change in practice: targeting individuals. *Int J Obes Relat Metab Disord.* 1996;20(Suppl 1):S22-S26.

I Am Often Asked About Bariatric Surgery. What Are the Different Weight Loss Surgeries for Pediatric Patients? What Are the Important Considerations, Associated Complications, and Effectiveness of Each Type of Surgery?

Stavra A. Xanthakos, MD, MS

When discussing weight loss surgery (WLS) options with your severely obese adolescent patient, it is important to understand and review the appropriate indications, the types of surgery available, and the associated risks and benefits. Adolescent patients should also be given realistic expectations about the degree of weight loss that can be anticipated with each type of surgery and an overview of the lifestyle changes they need to make to achieve long-term success. It is also helpful to identify WLS programs in your region that treat adolescent patients (including the age range they accept and the types of surgeries they offer to adolescents) and to ensure the program is adequately equipped to deal with the unique developmental needs of the adolescent patient. Such considerations include having staff adequately trained to work with adolescents and their family members, including adolescents who may have unique physical or mild developmental disabilities, as well as adolescent-appropriate support group offerings.[1] For example, we have treated severely obese adolescent patients in our program who have had mild developmental disability following resection of brain tumors (craniopharyngiomas) in early childhood and others who are wheelchair bound because of spina bifida.

Adolescent WLS is currently recommended for severely obese adolescents aged 13 to 19 years who have serious comorbid conditions and have failed to achieve significant and sustained weight loss through behavioral lifestyle changes alone (Table 34-1). These recommendations are based on available evidence of weight loss outcomes and comorbidity resolution and expert consensus opinion.[1] In addition, the adolescent should have reached skeletal and pubertal maturity (Tanner stage IV or V, and at least 95% of estimated linear growth) and have adequate family/social support. Adolescent patients may require more time than adult patients to become fully prepared for weight loss surgery and to completely understand its risks and benefits. The family or primary caretakers must be available to be actively involved in the preparation for surgery because most

Huang JS, ed. *Curbside Consultation in Pediatric Obesity: 49 Clinical Questions* (pp 155-160).
© 2014 Taylor & Francis Group

Table 34-1

Current Best Practice Recommendations for Considering Weight Loss Surgery in Severely Obese Adolescents[1]

Indications to Consider WLS in Adolescents With BMI ≥ 35 kg/m²

- Moderate to severe obstructive sleep apnea (apnea-hypopnea index > 15)
- Established type 2 diabetes mellitus
- Pseudotumor cerebri
- Severe and progressive nonalcoholic steatohepatitis

Indications to Consider WLS in Adolescents With BMI ≥ 40 kg/m²

- Cardiovascular disease risks (hypertension, dyslipidemia)
- Insulin resistance and impaired glucose tolerance
- Significantly impaired quality of life or activities of daily living
- Mild obstructive sleep apnea
- Mild nonalcoholic steatohepatitis

---

adolescents still live within a family unit and require family support to achieve success and adhere to recommendations. Absolute contraindications for WLS in adolescents include active untreated psychiatric disease, planned pregnancy in the next 1 to 2 years, and active substance abuse. It is also important to note that patients with Prader-Willi syndrome have been reported to have poor weight loss outcomes and a greater risk of complications compared with other severely obese adolescents and therefore are not considered good candidates for WLS.[2]

Appropriate adolescent candidates for WLS must also be able to provide informed consent/assent for surgery, have realistic expectations of weight loss, and should be willing to make at least a 6-month attempt to lose weight through a multidisciplinary weight loss program before surgery. This is important to ensure that the adolescent (1) has tried a rigorous medical weight loss program before committing to permanent surgical options because this rarely but occasionally results in sufficient weight loss that can improve comorbid conditions, (2) gains the lifestyle tools needed to maintain postoperative weight loss over the long term, and (3) ideally loses a small amount of weight (optimally up to 5%) before surgery to decrease liver size, which can improve operative access during surgery. Often insurance providers also require at least 6 months of documented participation in a medically supervised weight management program before they will approve an adolescent for weight loss surgery. Our surgical weight loss program offers a 6-month preoperative medical weight management program to candidates because many severely obese teens live in rural or isolated areas where they do not have access to a multidisciplinary weight loss program.

There are currently only 2 approved WLS options for adolescents: the Roux-en-Y gastric bypass (RYGB) and the sleeve gastrectomy (SG). The adjustable gastric band (AGB) is not approved by the US Food and Drug Administration (FDA) for patients younger than age 18 years. The RYGB (Figure 34-1A) is the current WLS gold standard with the most robust data on short- and long-term outcomes. In the RYGB procedure, the greater portion of the stomach is stapled off from the upper part of the stomach, leaving a 20- to 30-mL gastric pouch. The gastric pouch is then

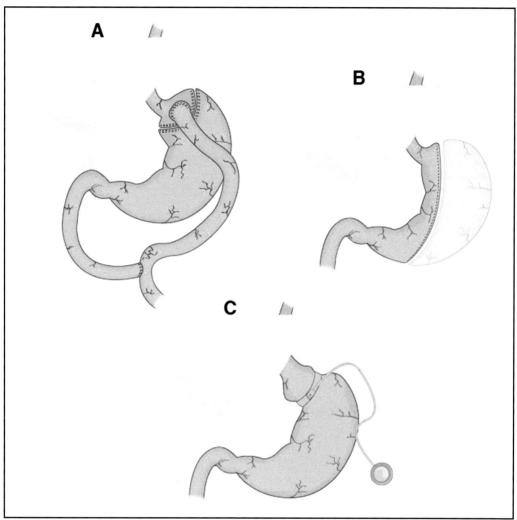

Figure 34-1. Most common types of weight loss surgery. (A) Roux-en-Y gastric bypass. (B) Sleeve gastrectomy. (C) Adjustable gastric band (not FDA approved for adolescents younger than 18 years of age).

anastomosed to a Roux-en-Y proximal jejunal segment, which bypasses the remaining stomach, duodenum, and a small portion of proximal jejunum. The typical Roux limb is 50 to 100 cm long, and the bypassed biliopancreatic limb is usually approximately 50 cm. The RYGB typically results in an approximately 35% mean body mass index (BMI) reduction in adolescents at 1-year postsurgery, regardless of the preoperative BMI.[3] Weight loss effects are believed to result from hormonal changes related to bypassing the stomach and first part of the small intestine, as well as restriction of dietary intake. Malabsorption is not believed to contribute significantly to weight loss, unless the Roux limb is longer (distal gastric bypass), which is uncommonly performed in adolescents. Perioperative risks of the RYGB include anastomotic leaks, anastomotic strictures, bowel obstruction, infection/sepsis, bleeding, and thromboembolic events. The rate of reoperations has been reported to be approximately 6.4% in a large series of 454 adolescent patients following RYGB.[4] No mortality has been reported to date in adolescents undergoing RYGB.

The SG (Figure 34-1B) was initially designed as the first part of a 2-stage weight loss procedure for extremely obese patients who were at high operative risk for a bypass procedure. In the

SG, the greater curvature of the stomach is stapled off and completely removed, leaving a slender longitudinal tube-shaped stomach that remains in continuity with the small bowel. This results in significant weight loss but with lower surgical risk. At a later stage after some weight has been lost, a small intestinal bypass procedure (either RYGB or biliopancreatic diversion/duodenal switch) would be performed as the definitive weight loss procedure. However, surgeons began to notice that adult patients undergoing SG experienced similar weight loss and comorbidity resolution compared with the RYGB, even up to 5 years postsurgery, leading to increased performance of SG as a stand-alone weight loss surgery in adults and more recently in adolescents as well. A large study of SG performed in 108 patients aged 5 to 21 years in Saudi Arabia reported good outcomes at 1 to 2 years postsurgery, with an approximately 30% BMI reduction, and comparable reduction in comorbid disease such as obstructive sleep apnea and diabetes.[5] Risks of SG are similar to those reported for RYGB, including gastric staple line leak, infection/sepsis, and bleeding. The rate of serious 30-day complications is low in adults at approximately 1%. Insufficient data are available at present to make accurate risk predictions for SG in adolescents. No serious complications were reported in a large series of pediatric patients undergoing SG in Saudi Arabia.[5]

Although the AGB is not FDA approved for adolescents younger than age 18 years, many adolescents inquire about this procedure because of the excellent perioperative safety profile (0.1% mortality rate in adults) and lower invasiveness of this procedure. The AGB (Figure 34-1C) involves implanting a ring-shaped silicone device with an adjustable balloon around the upper portion of the stomach, which creates a 30- to 50-mL gastric pouch just below the gastroesophageal junction. The balloon is connected by a catheter to a subcutaneous port. The diameter of the balloon can be increased or decreased by injecting or removing saline from the port, leading to varying degrees of dietary intake restriction due to early satiety. No bowel is bypassed, which reduces risk of nutritional complications. AGB can result in up to a 30% reduction in BMI in adolescents, with significant improvements in health status and quality of life, but typically the trajectory of weight loss is lower and requires frequent visits (on average 10 in the first year) for band adjustments to achieve maximal success. Long-term studies in adults suggest that the AGB results in significantly less weight loss than the RYGB over the long-term (5 to 10 years postoperatively). Complications of the AGB include band slippage, band erosions, band and port-site infections, port malposition, and esophageal dilations. Several recent studies have reported a relatively high rate of overall reoperations ranging from 8% to 15%, due to band-related complications. The AGB has not yet been approved by the FDA for adolescents but is still offered by some surgeons as an off-label procedure to adolescents after obtaining an investigational device exemption from the FDA. It is important to point out to adolescents that the AGB is not designed to be a reversible surgery and, with removal of the band, weight gain is likely to recur. Furthermore, even after removal, scar tissue would remain that can increase the technical difficulty of future weight loss surgeries.

The main long-term risk after all types of WLS are nutritional deficiencies related in part to inadequate intake and, in the case of RYGB, bypassing the duodenum and first portion of the jejunum. The most commonly reported nutritional deficiencies include iron, calcium, and vitamins D and B12. Lifelong nutritional supplements are recommended after all types of WLS (Table 34-2).[6] In the first 6 months after surgery, vitamin B1 is also recommended to reduce the risk of beriberi, which has been reported in the setting of excessive postoperative nausea and vomiting. Theoretically, the SG will be associated with reduced risk of deficiency due to lack of intestinal bypass, but there are insufficient long-term data on the prevalence of nutritional deficiencies after SG to guide specific reductions in supplements at this time. Reduction in acid production and intrinsic factor secretion likely also contribute to B12 deficiency after SG. All adolescents should be screened annually after WLS to identify nutritional deficiencies and correct them quickly. This is especially important for adolescent females of child-bearing age because nutritional deficiencies can also occur in infants of mothers who have severe nutritional deficiencies after WLS.

Table 34-2
Recommended Nutritional Supplements for Adolescents After Weight Loss Surgery

Recommended Micronutrient Supplementation After Weight Loss Surgery	
RYGB and sleeve gastrectomy	• Multivitamin with iron (100% to 200% of daily value) • Calcium citrate 1500 mg with vitamin D 1000 IU daily • B12: 500 µg sublingual daily or 1000 µg intramuscular monthly • Thiamine (B1): 50 mg orally daily (first 6 months) • Elemental iron 18 to 27 mg/day as needed in menstruating females or if anemia is present
Adjustable gastric band	• Multivitamin with iron (100% of daily value) • Calcium citrate 1500 mg with vitamin D 1000 IU daily • Thiamine (B1): 50 mg orally daily (first 6 months)
Recommended Nutritional Monitoring (Annually)	
Complete blood cell count with differential	
Serum iron, ferritin, transferring iron-binding capacity	
Serum vitamin 25 (OH) D, calcium, parathyroid hormone, alkaline phosphatase	
Serum vitamin B12 (cobalamin) and B1 (thiamine)	
Red blood cell folate	
Serum albumin and total protein	
Vitamin A (plasma retinol), E (plasma tocopherol), K (prothrombin time) after RYGB only	
Consider dual-energy X-ray absorptiometry to assess bone mineral density/content	

For females undergoing WLS, appropriate contraception should be offered for the first year after WLS because unexpected pregnancies can occur related to hormonal improvements in the menstrual cycle after weight loss. The levonorgestrel-releasing hormonal intrauterine device is an attractive option with an excellent safety profile and long-term (up to 5-year) yet easily reversible contraception with the ability to be implanted at the time of surgery. Overall, pregnancy risks (ie, preeclampsia, gestational diabetes) are reduced in adult females after WLS, but it is nonetheless recommended to avoid pregnancy in the first 18 months during the period of greatest weight loss.

Adolescent WLS is a tool that can produce significant and sustainable weight loss in severely obese adolescents with significant comorbid diseases. Several types of surgeries are available that have well-established weight loss outcomes and safety profiles in adults, with similarly positive data on safety and efficacy emerging in adolescent populations. The main long-term risks are micronutrient deficiencies. Lifelong adherence to micronutrient supplementation must be maintained to reduce the risk of nutritional complications.

References

1. Pratt JS, Lenders CM, Dionne EA, et al. Best practice updates for pediatric/adolescent weight loss surgery. *Obesity (Silver Spring).* 2009;17(5):901-910.
2. Scheimann AO, Butler MG, Gourash L, Cuffari C, Klish W. Critical analysis of bariatric procedures in Prader-Willi syndrome. *J Pediatr Gastroenterol Nutr.* 2008;46(1):80-83.
3. Inge TH, Jenkins TM, Zeller M, et al. Baseline BMI is a strong predictor of nadir BMI after adolescent gastric bypass. *J Pediatr.* 2010;156(1):103-108.
4. Treadwell JR, Sun F, Schoelles K. Systematic review and meta-analysis of bariatric surgery for pediatric obesity. *Ann Surg.* 2008;248(5):763-766.
5. Alqahtani AR, Antonisamy B, Alamri H, Elahmedi M, Zimmerman VA. Laparoscopic sleeve gastrectomy in 108 obese children and adolescents aged 5 to 21 years. *Ann Surg.* 2012;256(2):266-273.
6. Fullmer MA, Abrams SH, Hrovat K, et al. Nutritional strategy for adolescents undergoing bariatric surgery: report of a working group of the nutrition committee of NASPGHAN/NACHRI. *J Pediatr Gastroenterol Nutr.* 2012;54(1): 125-135.

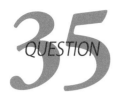

How Do I Get Reimbursed for Delivery of Weight Management Therapies in the Office?

Christopher F. Bolling, MD, FAAP

Although numerous strategies exist for weight management that show promise and large numbers of patients need and want help for managing weight, health care providers frequently are unable to provide weight management services because of challenges in getting reimbursed for labor-intensive and timely interventions. This chapter seeks to present a case for why and how financially viable weight management can be undertaken in a clinic setting.

The Case for In-Office Management

Several initiatives make pursuit of weight management in practice particularly urgent. Guidelines in 2007 from the American Academy of Pediatrics (AAP) laid out a detailed recommended approach for pediatricians to follow in their office to evaluate, prevent, and treat pediatric obesity.[1] Among these recommendations was one to treat obese patients with ongoing visits using counseling techniques such as motivational interviewing. In 2010, the National Commission on Quality Assurance made mandatory annual counseling by health care providers with their patients about weight status (body mass index [BMI] for adults and BMI percentile for age and sex for children), healthy nutrition, and physical activity.[2] In addition, various national organizations, including the Alliance for a Healthier Generation and the First Lady's Let's Move initiative, supported increased involvement of primary care providers in addressing obesity in the primary care setting.[3,4]

In addition to mandated and recommended activities, resources to prevent and treat obesity have rapidly multiplied. State programs like Let's Go from Maine (http://www.letsgo.org/), Ounce of Prevention/Pound of Cure from Ohio (http://ohioaap.org/projects/ounce-of-prevention/), and

Huang JS, ed. *Curbside Consultation in
Pediatric Obesity: 49 Clinical Questions* (pp 161-165).
© 2014 Taylor & Francis Group

Eat Smart Move More North Carolina (http://eatsmartmovemorenc.com/) provide localized and detailed approaches to obesity prevention and treatment. For reimbursement, national organizations such as the AAP Section on Obesity and the National Initiative on Children's Healthcare Quality Childhood Obesity Action Network provide effective programming and assistance with billing.

The mandate for providers is expansive. Providers are expected to practice prevention for all at the practice and community level, identify children at risk, provide ongoing therapy for the already obese, and efficiently refer the sickest and most severely affected patients. Of these complicated tasks, billing for ongoing counseling and therapy appears to be the most appropriate activities for traditional fee-for-service practice revenue generation. The other activities fall under standard practice expectations or "extracurricular" activities. Yet, these ongoing counseling visits are time consuming and potentially complicated, involving modification of a variety of behaviors, each of which is subject to variable patient motivation.

The Art of the Diagnosis and the Importance of Comorbidities

The history of weight management in medicine has been checkered. A lack of evidence and guidelines, the presence of numerous unproven (and often expensive) therapeutic modalities, and the perception that weight loss is a nonmedical, cosmetic issue have caused many insurers to not reimburse for or to specifically exclude treatment for obesity. As a result, charging for obesity services varies widely across the nation. Specifically, certain states discourage using the diagnostic codes for overweight and obesity by refusing payment if they are included, whereas others strongly encourage it by promoting statewide tracking and registries. The trend is definitely toward more clarity and transparency with increased use of these diagnoses.

The problematic use of the overweight and obesity codes makes the use of comorbidity codes extremely important in obtaining appropriate reimbursement (Table 35-1). An exhaustive history and physical are the keys for establishing more common comorbidities. Performing diagnostic testing to assess the presence of medical comorbidities relating to carbohydrate and lipid metabolism can also be a valuable strategy. Typically, one can use the Abnormal Weight Gain code initially until another comorbidity can be established. Abnormal values are more likely to be found as a patient ages but can be present even in young children. In extremely obese young children, sleep apnea is a common and serious comorbidity. For patients seen in tertiary obesity centers, care should be taken to ensure that comorbidity codes used do not compromise other referral clinics. For example, the obesity center may use Elevated Blood Pressure, whereas the preventive cardiology clinic uses Hypertension in certain institutions.

Strategies Around Codes

Evaluation and Management (E/M) codes are the workhorse codes for obesity care in the primary care clinic and are the most appropriate codes for use by physicians, nurse practitioners, and physician assistants. Brief (99211), Focused (99212), and Expanded (99213) codes are rarely appropriate because of the complex and timely nature of weight management. The multiple elements in the history (History of Present Illness, Review of Systems, and Family History in particular) and physical and the complex nature of medical decision making around multiple behaviors in the

Table 35-1
Diagnosis Codes

Primary Considerations	Others to Consider
278.00 Obesity, unspecified	Back, foot, and leg pain
278.01 Morbid (severe, >99th percentile BMI) obesity	Blount disease
	SCFE and Legg-Calvè-Perthes disease
278.02 Overweight	Shortness of breath
783.1 Abnormal weight gain	Wheezing
571.8 NAFLD or NASH	Obesity-hypoventilation syndrome
277.7 Hyperinsulinemia	PCOS
790.29 Hyperglycemia	Diabetes mellitus
272.4 Hyperlipidemia, not otherwise specified	Elevated glucose
	Thyroid disease
796.2 Elevated blood pressure	Abdominal pain
401 Hypertension	Headache
327.23 Sleep apnea, obstructive	Pseudotumor cerebri
701.2 *Acanthosis nigricans*	Polyphagia
307.50 Binge eating	Other dyslipidemias
307.59 Unspecified disorders of eating	Hypertension

Abbreviations: NASH, nonalcoholic steatohepatitis; NAFLD, nonalcoholic fatty liver disease; PCOS, polycystic ovarian syndrome; SCFE, slipped capital femoral epiphysis

obese/overweight child mean that initial visits are typically Comprehensive (99215) and follow-up visits are Detailed (99214).

A common pearl in billing is that "time trumps all," and this is true in weight management. Motivational interviewing–based counseling for weight management by definition is dictated by the patient's readiness to change. As such, the pace of change is variable and unique to each patient. Sessions take time and different patients take different amounts of time. Time spent in direct counseling must exceed 50% of the time displayed in Table 35-2. Be aware that complete documentation of History/Physical Examination/Medical Decision Making elements fulfilled and/or time spent is mandatory for reimbursement.

For practitioners in tertiary centers, the use of consultation codes closely mirrors use of E/M codes with Comprehensive (99245) used for initial visits and Detailed (99214) for most subsequent visits. Codes for prevention, group therapy, and counseling are often used by dietitians, health educators, and other allied professionals.

Table 35-2
Time-Based Coding for Established Patient

Visit Level	Time Requirement	50% Direct Face-to-Face Requirement (round up to nearest 5 minutes)
99211	5 minutes	5 minutes
99212	10 minutes	5 minutes
99213	15 minutes	10 minutes
99214	25 minutes	15 minutes
99215	40 minutes	20 minutes

Measurement and Quality Improvement

Quality improvement efforts in partnership with insurers also represent an opportunity for practices to be remunerated for obesity prevention and treatment. Obesity can be a useful tool for achieving and demonstrating improved outcomes. Specialty boards requiring proficiency in improvement science will often recognize efforts that improve screening of BMI percentile and efforts that document counseling for improved nutrition and activity. Intermediate outcomes such as these are obtainable and linked to ultimate improvement in children achieving a healthy weight.

Moving a measure like BMI should always be a goal, but weight loss across a community or other large population is influenced by many factors beyond the control of the medical provider. As more providers adopt practices that improve behaviors in their patients that are associated with healthy weight, there will be associated declines in obesity prevalence and severity as long as these practices are supported in other domains. However, demonstration of BMI reduction across even a practice population that is influenced by community, schools, state, and federal activities remains an elusive goal.

A Sample Case With Billing Recommendations

John Davis is a 12-year-old boy at Central Pediatric Clinic being seen by Dr. Smith for a well-child check. He is 5'2" and weighs 150 pounds with a normal blood pressure. This puts him at the 85th percentile for height, 98th percentile for weight, and 97th percentile for BMI. He has a strong family history for type II diabetes and is struggling to keep up with his friends in soccer because he says his back hurts excessively as the game wears on. He also says that other kids pick on him and challenge him repeatedly because of his size. He and his family say that they are very frustrated and are looking for ways to help John. John says that he wants to lose weight. Dr. Smith draws a thyroid-stimulating hormone test; liver function tests; hemoglobin A1c test; and fasting glucose, insulin, and lipid profile, and gives the family his number to set up a follow-up visit with him. **His well-child care visit is billed as a standard yearly check-up.** His labs are all normal except for an elevated fasting insulin of 24 mIU/L.

They come in to see you, Dr. Smith's partner, to discuss his labs and what to do next. You see them for 30 minutes explaining what labs were performed and what the elevated insulin level means and asking them for their reasons they want John to lose weight. They say they are ready to start a program. They decide to target John's excessive screen time. **You bill as a Comprehensive visit under the diagnoses of Hyperinsulinemia and Back Pain.**

John sees you 3 weeks later with no weight loss but good progress in reducing screen time to 1 hour per day. You reinforce this behavior and give the family several options on what behavior to pursue next, including appropriate portion size, eating a healthy breakfast, and eliminating sweet drinks. They pick the sweet drink goal. After discussing strategies to help them with this goal, **you bill as a Detailed visit with the diagnosis of Hyperinsulinemia.** The family sees you every 3 to 4 weeks to work on the other goals and to reinforce achieved goals. **You bill each visit as a Detailed visit with the same diagnosis**, and after 4 months John has demonstrated no weight gain and a ¾-inch height growth. They feel that they have a good routine going at this point and elect to follow up with you or Dr. Smith at his next check-up.

References

1. Barlow SE. Expert committee recommendations regarding the prevention, assessment, and treatment of child and adolescent overweight and obesity: summary report. *Pediatrics*. 2007;120(Suppl 4): S164-S192.
2. National Committee for Quality Assurance. HEDIS 2009 summary table of measures, product lines and changes. Washington, DC: Author; 2008. http://www.ncqa.org/HEDISQualityMeasurement/HEDISMeasures/HEDISArchives.aspx. Accessed April 25, 2009.
3. Rask KJ, Gazmararian JA, Kohler SS, Hawley JN, Bogard J, Brown VA. Designing insurance to promote use of childhood obesity prevention services, *J Obes*. 2013;2013: Article ID #379513. http://www.hindawi.com/journals/jobe/2013/379513/. Accessed December 6, 2013.
4. Executive Office of the President of the United States. Solving the Problem of Childhood Obesity in a Generation: White House Task Force on Childhood Obesity report to the President. Washington, DC: Author; 2010:33-36. http://www.letsmove.gov/sites/letsmove.gov/files/TaskForce_on_Childhood_Obesity_May2010_FullReport.pdf. Accessed December 6, 2013.

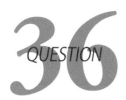

Are There Any Effective Technologies (Current Apps and Sensors) Available to Help Pediatric Patients Lose Weight?

Kevin Patrick, MD, MS

Background

The past decade has seen an unprecedented uptake of mobile phones and related technologies and their application to health-related issues—frequently called *mHealth*. MHealth applications are being developed and evaluated in adults for a variety of conditions, including asthma, smoking cessation, diabetes, obesity, stress, and depression. Although evidence of their overall effectiveness is limited, mobile access to health-related information and services is growing in importance, and an increasing proportion of health care services for people of all ages will be supported via mobile technologies. Recent national surveys indicate that 20% of Americans are using some form of technology to track an aspect of their health. Moreover, blending of the Web and mobile experience—the mobile Web—is happening at a rapid pace, and, importantly, is happening across essentially the entire socioeconomic spectrum, with many in mid-to-low–income communities using mobile devices more than computers for Web access. Thus, past research that demonstrates success with either Web- or mobile-based health interventions suggests promise for this integrated experience in the future.

In 2011, 95% of adolescents aged 12 to 17 years used the Internet and 77% owned cell phones. Web-based interventions for adolescents have been effective for the promotion of healthy eating and physical activity, and mHealth interventions have been used successfully to provide self-care tips and reminders to adolescents with diabetes to improve glycemic control. The greatest willingness to use online technology for health purposes has been reported among adolescents with chronic disease, and overweight adolescents endorse the use of technology to help them with weight-loss efforts. However, little research has been conducted to date in children or adolescents using mHealth strategies for obesity and obesity-related behaviors.

Huang JS, ed. *Curbside Consultation in Pediatric Obesity: 49 Clinical Questions* (pp 167-169).

Technologies Supported by mHealth That Can Be Leveraged for Obesity Treatment

MHealth technologies that are now in use to address obesity in people of all ages include text messaging or short messaging service (SMS, which works on all mobile phone types, not just smartphones); apps that reside on smartphones, increasingly the 2 predominant types being Apple's iOS and the Android platform developed by Google; and wearable devices such as pedometers or other types of separate accelerometer-based devices that capture walking and other forms of movement.

Short Messaging Service

Text messages, usually limited to 140 typed characters and sometimes also inclusive of a small graphic or picture, are in use worldwide. The popularity of SMS stems from its simplicity and ease of use, and SMS messages can be sent in a variety of languages. SMS messaging can support the delivery of tailored messaging, now considered a cornerstone of effective health behavior interventions. Moreover, they can go beyond simply "pushing" messages and provide interactive push/pull messaging to support ongoing tailoring based on the user's experience.

Text message–based interventions have been used to address a variety of health-related issues—from smoking to obesity to medication management—and SMS has been successfully used to address obesity in adults. Text messages show promise in addressing overweight behaviors in overweight children and obese adolescents at risk for type 2 diabetes and may also help support clinician counseling to improve weight-related parenting practices.

Mobile Apps

The growth in apps for smartphones has been extraordinary. Although smartphones incorporating some computer-like features have been around since the 1990s, it took the introduction of the Apple iPhone in 2007 to cause the marketplace to explode. The primary reason was the close coupling of the iPhone with the Apple iTunes platform that was already in wide use for downloading music to other Apple devices. Shortly thereafter, Google introduced the Android operating system and, unlike Apple, made it available to many handset developers. Now there are tens of thousands of apps available for both types of phones, and by mid-2013 Apple announced that 50 billion apps had been downloaded from their app store. As of March 2013, in the mHealth domain, 3 of the 5 most downloaded apps related to weight or weight-related behaviors, and weight loss was the single most popular category for content, almost double the second most popular, exercise (http://verasoni.com/mobile-health-applications-2012-study).

Although some of these apps may be targeted to children and adolescents, little to no published evidence exists of their effectiveness for weight loss in this population. Recent reviews of weight-related apps for adults have found limited evidence for how well they embody behavioral theory and evidence-based strategies for weight loss and their ultimate effectiveness. Thus, the field of apps for obesity treatment in childhood and adolescence is, as of this writing, still in its formative stage.

Wearable Health-Monitoring Devices

Wearable health-monitoring devices relevant to childhood obesity range from simple low-cost pedometers to accelerometer-based systems like Zamzee (HopeLab) that capture data from users to upload to a Web service that supports self-monitoring along with a game-like experience for children. Evidence is strong for the use of pedometers to promote improvements in physical activity in adults. Simply providing a patient with a pedometer has been shown to produce an increase of approximately 2000 steps/day over baseline and improve both BMI and blood pressure. Many adults find this form of self-monitoring activity to be enjoyable and something they can sustain over the long haul, and it is likely that some children and adolescents do as well. Pedometers are known to be effective in promoting physical activity in children and can promote increases in steps/day from 500 to 2500, in particular in those with low levels of activity. Pedometers come in a variety of types and price ranges, but no evidence exists that more expensive pedometers are more effective for general clinical use in terms of helping to promote activity. For children this can be important given the potential for loss and needed replacement.

A promising and evidence-based system available to promote improved physical activity in childhood is the Zamzee system. The system consists of an accelerometer-based device that can be clipped to a belt or elsewhere on the body that records activity for up to 2 weeks. Data from the device are uploaded via a USB port into a Web-based system where they can be tracked, shared with others, and used in game-like experience specifically attractive to children and early adolescents. In a study of middle school children using the device and website, moderate-to-vigorous physical activity (MVPA) increased an average of 59% over 1 week when compared with a control group and results were sustained for 6 months. A 27% increase in MVPA was also seen in overweight participants (BMI > 25) and a 103% increase in MVPA among girls.

Conclusion

Limited evidence exists for the efficacy of mobile phone–based apps and services and wearable health-monitoring devices to treat obesity in children and adolescents. However, the field of mHealth is growing rapidly in number and kinds of devices and sophistication of software to support them. Pediatricians, family physicians, and other health care providers who treat this population should monitor developments in this area and be prepared to leverage these increasingly ubiquitous technologies to address this compelling public health problem.

Suggested Readings

Bravata DM, Smith-Spangler C, Sundaram V, et al. Using pedometers to increase physical activity and improve health: a systematic review. *JAMA*. 2007;298(19):2296-2304.

Franklin VL, Greene A, Waller A, Greene SA, Pagliari C. Patients' engagement with "Sweet Talk"—a text messaging support system for young people with diabetes. *J Med Internet Res*. 2008;10(2):e20.

Lau PW, Lau EY, Wong del P, Ransdell L. A systematic review of information and communication technology-based interventions for promoting physical activity behavior change in children and adolescents. *J Med Internet Res*. 2011;13(3):e48.

Lubans DR, Morgan PJ, Tudor-Locke C. A systematic review of studies using pedometers to promote physical activity among youth. *Prev Med*. 2009;48(4):307-315.

Patrick K, Griswold WG, Raab F, Intille SS. Health and the mobile phone. *Am J Prev Med*. 2008;35(2):177-181.

Patrick K, Raab F, Adams MA, et al. A text message-based intervention for weight loss: randomized controlled trial. *J Med Internet Res*. 2009;11(1):e1.

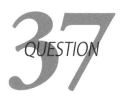

QUESTION

Sometimes Interventions That Do not Overtly Target Obesity (Stealth Interventions) Can Be Effective in Reducing Weight in Children. What Are Examples of Effective Stealth Interventions That Have Been Used for Reducing or Managing Weight in Childhood Obesity, and How Can We Better Use This Modality to Achieve Better Weight and Health in Children?

John R. Sirard, PhD and Jeanette M. Garcia, MS

It is no surprise to any health professional that pediatric obesity is a serious public health problem in the United States. Based on measured heights and weights obtained from the 2007-2008 National Health and Nutrition Examination Survey, 17% of the nation's youth aged 2 to 19 years, were classified as obese.[1] With the tragically high rate of pediatric obesity in the United States, it is clear that novel methods are needed to combat this epidemic. Unfortunately, it seems that one of the best ways to ensure that someone will *not* exercise or eat healthier is to tell him or her to exercise more and eat healthier. Research efforts to reverse the recent rise in pediatric obesity have often led to disappointing results.

The primary reason why traditional methods to improve physical activity and diet have proven insufficient, especially in youth, is that they emphasize outcome-based incentives for behavior change: reducing the risk of future chronic diseases. Such incentives have little, if any, tangible meaning for a young child. For adolescents, with their underdeveloped frontal lobe, feelings of invulnerability, and inability to see past next weekend's social activities, the concept of chronic disease prevention is a foreign concept for most.

A promising solution is the implementation of *stealth interventions*, a term coined by Dr. Tom Robinson from Stanford University's Lucille Packard School of Medicine.[2] The idea is to place the emphasis of the intervention on the *process* of behavior change rather than the outcomes. Therefore, a stealth intervention would focus on process motivators such as fun, social interaction/connection, and a sense of pride or accomplishment. These types of interventions promote intrinsic motivators such as enjoyment and self-confidence while producing the side effect of improved health. Another avenue by which stealth interventions work is through piggybacking onto existing social and ideological causes. Such causes or movements may have a greater appeal to children and promote a greater level of engagement and retention in our research and community-based

Huang JS, ed. *Curbside Consultation in Pediatric Obesity: 49 Clinical Questions* (pp 171-173).
© 2014 Taylor & Francis Group

programs while fostering a healthy lifestyle change. A few examples of stealth interventions are worth a closer look.

One interesting example is the use of ethnic dance for African American and Hispanic girls as a means of preserving cultural identity, providing social interaction in a safe environment, and most important, having fun. In an early pilot study, boys and girls were randomized into either a dance group or a standard physical education (PE) class.[3] The results indicated that girls who participated in the dance group had a significantly lower body mass index (BMI) and resting heart rate (a measure of aerobic fitness) than girls in the standard PE class. No significant changes were observed for the boys. It was concluded that the dance class was fun and interesting to girls, therefore providing intrinsic motivation to engage in the activity. These findings were of great importance considering that few PE interventions have shown any improvement in body composition.[4] The findings from the Flores[3] study led to the implementation of dance classes that emphasized immediate motivators such as enjoyment and pride in cultural heritage, rather than end-result outcomes such as weight loss. The subsequent Stanford Girls Health Enrichment Multi-site Studies project implemented a similar type of ethnic dance intervention on a larger scale.[5] A decreased rate of weight gain resulted for the girls in the dance intervention (which also included a TV reduction component) but by the end of the study, the intervention and control groups did not differ significantly in BMI.

Improved health benefits may also be a side effect of social movements and policies,[2] a method that is only beginning to be realized. For example, individuals who are passionate about preserving the environment (sustainability, climate change, going green) may attempt to reduce their carbon footprint by using automobiles less and engaging more frequently in walking or riding a bicycle. Thus, an increase in physical activity and health is a side effect of an individual's environmental stewardship, not the main outcome. For children, this may be accomplished via walk-to-school initiatives[6] and park and trail clean-up days—performed in the name of environmentalism but with increased physical activity as an additional benefit.

Similarly, school and community gardens have become increasingly popular as a means of introducing children to healthy fruits and vegetables. A side effect of such gardening activities is an increase in physical activity associated with digging, weeding, watering, and other basic gardening tasks. Although this may not always be high-intensity activity, the work performed in the garden could amount to a significant increase in daily physical activity for many sedentary children. Research evidence supports the use of school gardens as a means of getting children to try new fruits and vegetables, increase regular consumption of fruits and vegetables, and gain experience in preparing healthy food.[7] Here, too, environmentalism can be leveraged by promoting organic growing methods. An additional benefit of school gardens is the ability to tie in academic subject material (math, science, reading), providing an experiential learning opportunity with far-reaching academic and health outcomes. What to do with the bounty that the school garden produces? Feed the school, feed the needy, start a farm stand, sell at a local farmer's market, or the children can take those organically grown goodies home, where they can help Mom or Dad in the kitchen. Cooking with a child can be challenging, but it is a fun activity for children, provides a way to spend some quality time with Mom and Dad, and fosters social support for healthier eating by getting the whole family involved. To a child, the school garden can be fun and intrinsically motivating. The child gets out of the classroom and digs in the dirt, takes pride in making something grow and transform from seed to dinner table, and becomes more confident in his or her ability to grow, eat, and prepare healthy food—and we also worked in a healthy dose of physical activity along the way. Similarly, a child who is passionate about animal rights may abstain from or reduce his or her meat consumption. Eating this way is adopted not for the health benefits, but a diet high in vegetables, fruits, and whole grains will provide healthy side effects such as a lower BMI and reduced risk factors for heart disease and type 2 diabetes.

Mentoring programs also provide a way to sneak in messages related to physical activity and diet. There is an emerging body of literature on the health benefits of adult-youth mentoring programs. In a recent study of mentoring in African American teenagers,[8] the authors observed improvements in some dietary variables, body composition, and weight status after 2 years of follow-up. Another study observed beneficial changes in adolescent eating behaviors after a similar mentoring program.[9] Although not a stealth intervention per se, the ability to use such ubiquitous mentoring programs to reach and improve the lives of many young people academically, socially, and also physically appears to be a promising avenue for future research and community-based programming.

Finally, stealth interventions can be designed around the natural and built environment that we inhabit. For example, installing new lighting and building or repairing sidewalks, crosswalks, and crosswalk signals can provide a safer environment for pedestrians but are likely to be driven by a desire to decrease neighborhood crime rates. Downtown revitalization projects may be initiated to improve safety, economic vitality, and aesthetics, but they should also include design elements that support multiple types of healthy physical activity like pedestrian facilities, playgrounds, and cycling lanes or paths that can link to other neighborhoods, trails, or recreation facilities.

There are numerous ways that physical activity and diet can be surreptitiously inserted into children's routines while they are blissfully unaware that they have taken a step toward a healthier future. Getting a child to adopt a healthier lifestyle doesn't have to mean constant lectures of how the child should be active to stave off cardiovascular disease and diabetes while watching his or her eyes glaze over. By emphasizing the process (and the fun) of the behaviors and building on an existing interest or social cause, improvements in health become an ancillary benefit of the process. Allied health professionals are concerned with chronic disease. Children are concerned with having fun. The stealth intervention technique could help meet both goals and help children develop habits that will carry over into adulthood.

References

1. Ogden CL, Carroll MD, Kit BK, Flegal KM. Prevalence of obesity and trends in body mass index among US children and adolescents, 1999-2010. *JAMA*. 2012;307(5):483-490.
2. Robinson TN. Save the world, prevent obesity: piggybacking on existing social and ideological movements. *Obesity (Silver Spring)*. 2010;18(Suppl 1):S17-S22.
3. Flores R. Dance for health: improving fitness in African American and Hispanic adolescents. *Public Health Rep*. 1995;110(2):189-193.
4. Harris KC, Kuramoto LK, Schulzer M, Retallack JE. Effect of school-based physical activity interventions on body mass index in children: a meta-analysis. *CMAJ*. 2009;180(7):719-726.
5. Robinson TN, Matheson DM, Kraemer HC, et al. A randomized controlled trial of culturally tailored dance and reducing screen time to prevent weight gain in low-income African American girls: Stanford GEMS. *Arch Pediatr Adolesc Med*. 2010;164(11):995-1004.
6. Sirard JR, Slater ME. Walking and bicycling to school: a review. *Am J Lifestyle Med*. 2008;2(5):372-396.
7. Knai C, Pomerleau J, Lock K, McKee M. Getting children to eat more fruit and vegetables: a systematic review. *Prev Med*. 2006;42(2):85-95.
8. Black DS, Grenard JL, Sussman S, Rohrbach LA. The influence of school-based natural mentoring relationships on school attachment and subsequent adolescent risk factors. *Health Education Research*. 2010;25(5):892-902.
9. Haire-Joshu D, Nanney MS, Elliott M, et al. The use of mentoring programs to improve energy balance behaviors in high-risk children. *Obesity (Silver Spring)*. 2010;18(Suppl 1):S75-S83.

QUESTION 38

WHAT ARE PARENT-ONLY INTERVENTIONS FOR CHILDHOOD OBESITY, AND ARE THEY EFFECTIVE?

Kerri N. Boutelle, PhD and Stephanie Knatz, PhD

The current empirically supported treatment for childhood obesity is behavioral family-based treatment (FBT). FBT involves parents as well as children and includes nutrition education, exercise, and behavior therapy techniques. Data suggest that one-third of children who participate in this program are no longer overweight in adulthood.[1] Here we describe the data on parent-only treatments for childhood obesity, then describe the key components of FBT and how these can be applied by parents without their children's involvement.

What Are Parent-Only Treatments?

Parent-only treatments for childhood obesity provide all of the education and skills needed to assist a child with weight loss to the parent alone, without the attendance of the child. Parent-only treatments are used to deliver treatments for other child behavioral issues, including tantrums, self-destructive behaviors, verbal aggression, excessive crying, thumb sucking, school phobia, and oppositional behavior, and can naturally be applied to obesity as well. Parents are the most important people in a child's environment and are primarily responsible for reinforcing and supporting the acquisition and maintenance of eating and exercise behaviors. Typically, these skills have been taught to parents in classes. However, these skills could also be taught in a medical clinic or in other community settings.

Parent-only programs provide education on dietary and physical activity requirements necessary to achieve weight loss. In addition, these programs teach the core behavior therapy strategies to treat childhood obesity, including teamwork, specificity regarding behavior, self-monitoring, goal setting, stimulus control, and positive parenting strategies.[2] These strategies are described in more detail later in this chapter.

Huang JS, ed. *Curbside Consultation in Pediatric Obesity: 49 Clinical Questions* (pp 175-178).

Parent-only treatments are of interest because they are less expensive to deliver than parent and child treatments[3] and offer greater opportunities for dissemination because the meetings do not have to coordinate around both parent and child schedules. In addition, it is developmentally appropriate to deliver the majority of skills directly to the parents because they are responsible for the majority of food preparation and purchasing and for providing opportunities for physical activity. Parent-only treatments may be more appropriate for children who are shy, have behavioral problems, or are ashamed to attend behavioral weight loss groups.

Data on Parent-Only Treatments for Childhood Obesity

The published data on parent-only treatments for childhood obesity suggest that parent-only treatments are a viable alternative to parent and child treatments. In a randomized, controlled trial, we showed that parent-only treatments resulted in similar weight loss to parent and child treatments immediately after treatment and 6 months after treatment.[4] Furthermore, in a study with rural families, both parent-only and family-based interventions resulted in significant weight loss compared with a no-treatment control group, even at 10 months after treatment.[5]

To date, the majority of these studies have focused on children aged 12 years and younger. For youth aged older than 13 years, few data exist on parent-only treatments, and use of these programs should be approached cautiously. When working with teens, the developmental age of the child should be taken into account, and the model should be more collaborative between parents and teen. However, even older teens still need parents to assist them with some behavioral management skills and can benefit from parental support.

Key Parenting Components for Family-Based Treatment

Teamwork

It is important that parents work on changing their own eating and physical activity behavior along with their children. Most parents can work on improving their eating and increasing their physical activity for health reasons, even parents who are not overweight. This sense of teamwork will make a child a more willing participant, and changes won't feel as negative. In fact, working on changing these hard behaviors together can strengthen parent-child relationships. One of the best predictors of child weight loss is parent weight loss,[6] so a parent's participation in changing his or her own behaviors can assist the child in weight loss.

Specificity

Identification of specific behaviors to be changed by obese youth and their parents is an initial step for behavior change. Rather than recommending nonspecific changes, such as "lose weight," "eat less," or "exercise more," it is important for parents to identify specific behaviors for change. For example, "This week, let's exercise at the gym 3 days a week for 1 hour," or "We will commit to track our food intake 4 out of 7 days this week." Selection of target behaviors can be decided by the parents or the obese youth, but ideally these decisions should be made in collaboration.

SELF-MONITORING

Once target behaviors have been identified, self-monitoring of those behaviors is important. Self-monitoring refers to keeping track of food, physical activity, and weight by recording these behaviors on a regular basis. Keeping track of these behaviors is important to evaluate progress toward goals and to change behavior accordingly. Self-monitoring can be as simple as writing down what one eats, keeping a weight chart, or tracking eating and physical activity using a paper chart or a number of Internet-based tracking applications. Self-monitoring is a reliable predictor of weight loss in obese children and adults. Parents can discuss self-monitoring and can self-monitor with their children using any of the methods described previously.

GOAL SETTING

Setting daily or weekly specific goals for changing behavior is important to evaluate success in weight loss programs. Smaller, achievable goals at first are considered important to develop self-confidence and decrease frustration. It is important to set both short- and long-term goals. Adjusting goals is an ongoing process that requires a parent's attention.

STIMULUS CONTROL

Stimulus control refers to structuring the home environment to make it healthier and easier for the child to eat fewer calories and exercise more. It is important for parents to remove most, if not all, high-calorie foods and to increase the availability of fruits and vegetables and healthier options. Other recommendations include restricting eating locations in the home (only at the dinner table or island), not having television in the children's bedrooms, relocating snacks to be less visible, portioning food before serving, restricting eating in front of the television, using smaller dinnerware, and reducing visits to restaurants or fast food. Stimulus control can also be used to promote physical activity, such as having exercise balls in the home and other physically interactive games and activities. Starting traditions that include physical activity can be good for the whole family. All of these stimulus-control strategies can be implemented by the parent at home without engaging the child.

Positive Reinforcement Strategies

Parents are able to help their children more than they think. Discussions regarding weight loss are often negative, focusing on what the child is not doing right. The use of praise and reinforcement by parents is an incredible behavior change tool that is often underused. Positive reinforcement strategies include praise and child recognition, as well as time spent together and rewards/prizes (that do not involve money or food). Parents need to recognize that most children do not want to be overweight and that catching their child doing something for the program is one of the most important ways they can help their child change their behavior. Let's use the example of going to a birthday party and having one piece of pizza. Some parents would criticize the child for having the pizza, but changing their response to praising the child for not having 2 pieces of pizza is important to shape the child's behavior and to improve the parent-child relationship around weight-related issues. These types of parenting skills can often take practice, and engaging partners to help in the process of using a positive reinforcement can be useful to make changes.

In addition, many programs use a formal reinforcement system (motivation system) by which the child earns points for program-related behaviors. Behaviors that might qualify include self-monitoring, exercise, lifestyle exercise, meeting weight loss goals, and reducing high-fat, high-calorie food intake. Parents and their children can set up a point system based on these behaviors and then identify small, medium, and large rewards that the children can trade their points in for. The most important part of this kind of program is to make sure that the points are allotted and discussed on a regular basis. Because making physical activity and eating changes can be challenging for youth, a point system that incorporates rewards that the child is willing to work for can enhance internal motivation.

Challenges to Engaging Parents in a Parent-Only Treatment

Although the studies on parent-only treatments suggest that working solely with parents will produce results that are similar or even better than working with parents and children, some parents will not believe in their own ability to assist their children with weight loss. They might make comments about their child's motivations or laziness. They might make comments about someone needing to "talk the child into doing this" or say that they have tried everything. Instead of being dissuaded by these comments, providers can spend some time with the parent discussing and improving their self-efficacy. Children may seem lazy or unmotivated, but most children who are overweight would like to change and may be receptive to their parents providing structure around eating and physical activity to help them. Often parents need to be convinced of this, but the data suggest that they can do it. Even if the child isn't a willing participant, parents still have the ability to engage in most of the previously mentioned skills without the collaboration of the child. This can often be challenging, but when it is discussed with the child, it can be put in the context of, "I'm doing this because I love you and want you to be healthy."

Conclusion

Parents play a significant role in assisting their children in losing weight. Many parenting skills can be implemented with or without the child's collaboration, and studies on parent-only treatments show that the outcomes are as good as or even better than parent and child treatments.

References

1. Epstein LH, Valoski A, Wing RR, McCurley J. Ten-year outcomes of behavioral family-based treatment for childhood obesity. *Health Psychol*. 1994;13(5):373-383.
2. Faith MS, Van Horn L, Appel LJ, et al. Evaluating parents and adult caregivers as "agents of change" for treating obese children: evidence for parent behavior change strategies and research gaps: a scientific statement from the American Heart Association. *Circulation*. 2012;125(9):1186-1207.
3. Janicke DM, Sallinen BJ, Perri MG, Lutes LD, Silverstein JH, Brumback B. Comparison of program costs for parent-only and family-based interventions for pediatric obesity in medically underserved rural settings. *J Rural Health*. 2009;25(3):326-330.
4. Boutelle KN, Cafri G, Crow SJ. Parent-only treatment for childhood obesity: a randomized controlled trial. *Obesity (Silver Spring)*. 2011;19(3):574-580.
5. Janicke DM, Sallinen BJ, Perri MG, et al. Comparison of parent-only vs family-based interventions for overweight children in underserved rural settings: outcomes from project STORY. *Arch Pediatr Adolesc Med*. 2008; 162(12):1119-1125.
6. Boutelle KN, Cafri G, Crow SJ. Parent predictors of child weight change in family based behavioral obesity treatment. *Obesity (Silver Spring)*. 2012;20(7):1539-1543.

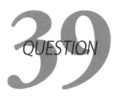

WHAT PUBLIC POLICIES HAVE BEEN EFFECTIVE FOR THE PREVENTION OF CHILDHOOD OBESITY?

Sandra Hassink, MD, FAAP

The socioecological model has been used to capture the multiple individual, familial, social, cultural, and economic influences on the obesity epidemic. In 2001, the *Surgeon General's Call to Action to Prevent and Decrease Overweight and Obesity*[1] recognized the importance of a public health response. It is clear that obesity is one of our most important pediatric public health problems and as such demands solutions based both on individual- and population-level change.

The Institute of Medicine (IOM) report *Accelerating Progress in Obesity Prevention*[2] recommended that a multisector strategy be used so that changes encouraging healthy eating and activity occur in school environments, food and beverage environments, health care and work environments, and physical activity environments with an overarching approach to a population-based healthy message environment. The IOM also encouraged people to increase their level of engagement in whatever venues to which they have access to improve nutrition and activity environments and options.

One important evidence-based framework for working with communities to develop public policies/strategies to have a positive effect on population health is that of the MAPPS strategies.[3] These strategies include Media, Access, Point of decision information, Price, and Social support/services. States and communities have found these to be effective points of intervention, and they are used by the Centers for Disease Control (CDC) in the Communities Putting Prevention to Work grantee communities.[4] The MAPPS strategies are applied to nutrition and physical activity in Tables 39-1 and 39-2.

The following are some examples of community-level nutrition strategies that have been put into place:

- In Seattle, retailers located in food deserts were provided incentives to offer fresh fruit and vegetables. Demand increased, and residents now have greater access to healthy foods.

Huang JS, ed. *Curbside Consultation in Pediatric Obesity: 49 Clinical Questions* (pp 179-182).

Table 39-1
MAPPS Strategies to Support Changes in Nutrition

Media	• Advertise restrictions on unhealthy foods • Promote healthy foods and drinks • Address counter-advertising of unhealthy foods
Access	• Increase access to healthy foods and drinks • Limit access to unhealthy foods and drinks • Reduce density of fast food establishments • Limit trans fat consumption through standards, labeling, and purchasing • Reduce sodium consumption through standards, labeling, and purchasing • Address food procurement and purchasing processes • Support farm-to-institution food supply
Point of Purchase/ Promotion	• Signage for healthy and less-healthy food items • Menu labeling • Product placement and attractiveness
Price	• Change relative prices of healthy and unhealthy items
Social Support and Services	• Support breastfeeding through policy change and maternal care practices

---

- The San Diego school district connected local farms with public schools in a farm-to-school lunch program providing access to fresh food to local school children.

  Some examples of successful community strategies include the following:

- Jefferson County, Alabama, strengthened local school wellness policies to include a physical activity requirement for all elementary school students. All students in kindergarten through 5th grade were required to participate in 30 minutes of daily physical activity.

- La Crosse County, Wisconsin, added 6 miles of bike lanes to city streets, quadrupling the number of available bike lanes.

  Legislation and public policies have also been instrumental in obesity prevention. State-level legislative efforts have been ongoing and have focused on schools by taking the following actions:

- Improving standards for school meals (see Healthy Hunger-Free Kids Act on p. 181)

- Reducing competitive foods

- Screening body mass index (BMI)

- Adding or increasing nutrition education

- Adding or increasing physical education

- Promoting farm-to-school programs

Table 39-2

MAPPS Strategies to Support Changes in Physical Activity

Media	• Promote increased physical activity • Promote use of public transit • Promote activity transportation (walking and biking) • Counter-advertising for screen time
Access	• Create safe, attractive, accessible places for activity • City planning and zoning that supports physical activity • Require daily quality physical education in schools • Require daily quality physical activity in after-school and child care • Restrict screen time in after-school and child care
Point of Purchase/ Promotion	• Signage for walkable neighborhood destinations • Signage for public transportation
Price	• Reduced price for park and facility use • Incentive for active transit • Subsidize membership to recreational facilities
Social Support and Services	• Safe routes to school • Workplace, faith, neighborhood, park activity groups

- Increasing school recess
- Implementing obesity prevention in school wellness policies
- Creating joint use agreements for school facilities
- Implementing preschool obesity prevention

Other state legislation has included the following actions:

- Instituting complete streets laws
- Placing sales taxes on sodas
- Creating tax exemptions and tax credits to increase fresh food access
- Menu labeling
- Mandating diabetes screening and education

The Healthy Hunger-Free Kids Act (2010) requires the US Department of Agriculture to establish nutrition standards for school meals and all food sold in schools. New standards for school meals include (1) ensuring students are offered fruits and vegetables every day of the week; (2) substantially increasing offerings of whole grain–rich foods; (3) offering only fat-free or low-fat milk varieties; (4) limiting calories based on the age of children being served to ensure proper portion size; and (5) increasing the focus on reducing the amounts of saturated fat, trans fats, and sodium.

How Do Pediatricians Get Involved?

For the busy practitioner, it may seem daunting to get involved in community-based change. The American Academy of Pediatrics has created a Policy Tool online (http://www2.aap.org/obesity/matrix_1.html)[5] that is geared to help practitioners make the transition from practice to policy. These tools take the familiar points of intervention used clinically in obesity prevention and treatment 5210 (ie, 5 fruits and vegetables, 2 hours of screen time, 1 hour of physical activity, 0 sugar-sweetened beverages) along with breastfeeding and BMI, and connects them to the MAPPS strategies applicable to the practice, school, community, state, and federal levels.

Each cell showcases the following:

- Policy opportunities and possible action steps at various levels (eg, community, school)
- Organizations recommending the policy strategies (eg, IOM, CDC)
- Links to additional resources

Links to Relevant Data Sources

This allows the practitioner to find interventions and resources suited to the venue in which he or she is working. Once a policy option has been chosen, the practitioner can work to (1) increase recognition of the problem; (2) compile evidence, data, and stories that illustrate the problem from multiple dimensions; (3) identify strategies that address the problem; and (4) be alert for windows of opportunity such as timing of legislations, the appearance of a policy champion, working with personal connections, and/or the occurrence of a focusing event. Pediatricians can be powerful advocates in their communities, with their families and patients, and in their own offices. They are key to highlighting the need to continue to focus both on obesity prevention and treatment.

Some evidence exists of slowing and/or stabilizing the increase in obesity rates,[6] and although time is needed to confirm this trend, it is possible that public health efforts and campaigns may be starting to have an effect. Nevertheless, current rates remain at high levels, and continued multisector intervention is needed at the individual, family, community, state, and federal levels.[7]

References

1. US Department of Health and Human Services. *The Surgeon General's Call To Action To Prevent and Decrease Overweight and Obesity 2001*. Rockville, MD: US Department of Health and Human Services, Public Health Service, Office of the Surgeon General; 2001. http://www.surgeongeneral.gov/library/calls/obesity/CalltoAction.pdf.pdf. Accessed November 12, 2013.
2. Institute of Medicine. *IOM 2012 Accelerating Progress in Obesity Prevention Solving the Weight of the Nation*. Washington, DC: The National Academic Press; 2012.
3. US Department of Health and Human Services, Centers for Disease Control and Prevention. MAPPS interventions for communities putting prevention to work. 2001. http://www.cdc.gov/chronicdisease/recovery/PDF/MAPPS_Intervention_Table.pdf. Accessed November 12, 2013.
4. Centers for Disease Control and Prevention. Communities putting prevention to work. http://www.cdc.gov/nccdphp/dch/programs/CommunitiesPuttingPreventiontoWork/. Accessed November 12, 2013.
5. American Academy of Pediatrics. Policy Opportunities Tool. http://www2.aap.org/obesity/matrix_1.html. Accessed November 12, 2013.
6. Trust for America's Health and Robert Wood Johnson Foundation. *F as in Fat: How Obesity Threatens America's Future*. Washington, DC: Trust for America's Health; 2012.
7. National Conference of State Legislators. Childhood obesity: 2011 update of legislative policy options. http://www.ncsl.org/issues-research/health/childhood-obesity-2011.aspx. Accessed November 12, 2013.

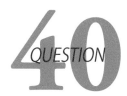

WHAT DO I NEED TO ACCOMMODATE THE OBESE CHILD AND FAMILY IN THE CLINICAL OFFICE IN REGARD TO FURNITURE AND EQUIPMENT?

Victor E. Uko, MD, MRCPCH (UK) and Kimberly P. Newton, MD

The relatively high prevalence of obesity among children and adults, coupled with the prevalence of accompanying comorbidities, implies that a significant number of obese patients will visit the clinical office and seek access to health care services. It is imperative that the clinical office is designed to make adequate provisions in order to create a welcoming and conducive atmosphere for the delivery of effective care to the obese child and members of his or her family.

When planning a welcoming setting for patients, the social environment must be considered in addition to the physical environment. The social and emotional challenges faced by obese and overweight individuals are often ignored. The stigma, bias, and subtle discrimination encountered by this group of patients in the current health care climate can be damaging to both their emotional and physical health.[1] The perceptions that the obese patient is lazy, lacking in self-control, and unintelligent are some of the negative attitudes that are often portrayed by health care providers.[2] Research has shown that this weight bias shown by health care providers, combined with the embarrassment sometimes faced by obese patients (eg, while being weighed) leads these patients to avoid seeking medical services. Therefore, it is important to create a conducive and welcoming environment for all patients, including the obese child and his or her family members, starting with the education of all office personnel. Opportunities for weight-related sensitivity training, along with other training schemes that address patient diversity and culture, should be made available to all health care providers. For example, a resource that may be used for such purposes is the Yale Rudd Center for Food Policy and Obesity, which offers an online toolkit and training modules for health care providers.[3]

The recurrent office visits by the obese population may be better tolerated by reducing certain physical barriers or limitations that may be present in the office setting. The ingress and egress of the obese child and family members when visiting the clinical office should be an important consideration in the overall office design and layout. Providing appropriately sized wheelchairs at the entrance to the clinic is a simple first step to accommodate those with hip or ambulatory issues.

Huang JS, ed. *Curbside Consultation in Pediatric Obesity: 49 Clinical Questions* (pp 183-184).
© 2014 Taylor & Francis Group

If physician input is accepted in the design phase of building a clinical office space, then particular attention should be paid to the architectural design of the hallways, elevators, and toilet facilities. The entry points to the buildings should have comfortable ramps with handrails, and doors should have a minimum width of 3 feet, 2 inches.[4] The elevators should have the capacity to accommodate patients transported in wheelchairs and, on rare occasions, in hospital beds. The toilets should also have a wide door width, floor-mounted seats, and strong grab bars for support.[5] The waiting and registration area in the clinician's office is often the first place patients and their families are received. It is thus important that the furniture and design of this area cater to all patient groups, especially the obese child and his or her family members. Providing a mix of furniture suitable for the obese population is advisable. Armless chairs, loveseats, and seating benches with appropriate weight limits are examples of furniture that are amenable to this group of patients. The Americans with Disabilities Act and Section 504 of the Rehabilitation Act are 2 pieces of federal legislation that govern equal access to health care services for individuals with disabilities and thus provide an important legal impetus for ensuring availability of appropriate facilities for all individuals, including those who may be obese.

The medical equipment used during clinical visits should also accommodate the obese child and adult family members. This includes examination tables and chairs that have the appropriate size and weight capacity. The examination tables should ideally be height adjustable with a minimum height of 17 to 19 inches from the floor to the top of the cushion to facilitate easy lateral transfer of patients in wheelchairs. The table's cushion top should be extra wide (24 inches or more) with a weight capacity of at least 400 pounds to accommodate patients of all sizes. Scales should be used that have a capacity range of at least 500 to 800 pounds to accurately measure the largest pediatric patients, especially those who may need to be weighed in a wheelchair. The weighing scales should also be placed in a relatively private area that will allow staff to discreetly obtain weights free of judgment or commentary because this may be a sensitive issue for obese patients. Other equipment such as large blood pressure cuffs (adult- and thigh-sized), measuring tapes, and appropriately sized gowns that fit the habitus of the obese child should be readily available in the clinician's office. Provisions also need to be made for obese patients who may require additional evaluation, such as laboratory or radiological tests at the clinician's office. The phlebotomy area should have armless chairs and benches similar to those provided in the waiting areas. If at all possible, modifications should be made to the diagnostic imaging equipment (such as ultrasound probes, computed tomography/magnetic resonance imaging tubes, and other conventional radiology equipment as deemed necessary) to accommodate the size and habitus of the obese patient. Clinicians also should inquire about the weight capacity and size limitations of imaging machines in their local communities to help with appropriate referrals as needed.

It is imperative that weight-based sensitivity training for health care providers along with the provision of appropriate facilities and equipment for easy accessibility remain central to the design of the clinical office. These are necessary components required for the delivery of quality health care, the provision of an inclusive environment, and the adherence to some of the legislative requirements for the care of individuals handicapped by such limitations as their overall weight and size.

References

1. Puhl R, Brownell KD. Bias, discrimination, and obesity. *Obes Res.* 2001;9(12):788-805.
2. Puhl RM, Brownell KD. Confronting and coping with weight stigma: an investigation of overweight and obese adults. *Obesity (Silver Spring).* 2006;14(10):1802-1815.
3. Yale Rudd Center for Food Policy and Obesity. Preventing weight bias: helping without harming in clinical practice. http://www.yaleruddcenter.org/what_we_do.aspx?id=10. Accessed January 6, 2013.
4. Collignon A. Strategies for accommodating obese patients in an acute care setting. *AAH.* http://www.aia.org/groups/aia/documents/pdf/aiab090823.pdf. Updated November 22, 2010. Accessed January 12, 2013.
5. Andrade SD. Planning and design guidelines for bariatric healthcare facilities. *AAAH.* http://www.aia.org/groups/aia/documents/pdf/aiab090827.pdf. Updated November 22, 2010. Accessed January 12, 2013.

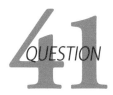

DO I DOSE MEDICATIONS THE SAME FOR AN OBESE CHILD AS FOR A NORMAL WEIGHT CHILD?

Jennifer Le, PharmD, MAS, BCPS-ID, FCCP, FCSHP

Understanding general pharmacokinetic alterations stemming from physiological changes that occur with age as well as obesity are crucial to optimize drug dosing in obese children, especially in light of limited pharmacokinetic studies.[1] This chapter will review body fat measurements and basic pharmacokinetic alterations that occur with age and obesity.

Measurements of Body Fat

Although possessing minimal metabolic activity, excessive amounts of adipose tissue, as in the case of obesity, significantly affect body size that may consequently alter drug pharmacokinetics and dosing. A reliable measurement of body fat is necessary for accurate drug dosing. Indirect measures of body composition are often used to classify the degree of obesity (ie, overweight or obese) and are commonly used for pediatric drug dosing.[1] These indirect methods are inexpensive and convenient because they are derived from a patient's height, weight, or girth, all of which are easily measured by the clinician. These measures include body mass index (BMI), body surface area (BSA), ideal body weight (IBW), and adjusted body weight (AdjBW; Table 41-1).

The Centers for Disease Control uses BMI to categorize the degree of obesity in children and adolescents. BMI varies by sex and age, with values slightly higher in girls than boys and a steady increase from age 5 to 7 years. Although BMI correlates well to adiposity, it does not account for high lean body mass (eg, as observed in some male adolescents). It is also excessively sensitive to stature variation, with tall adolescents appearing to be erroneously obese.

BSA is most commonly used for the dosing of chemotherapeutic agents in children. Similar to BMI, BSA incorporates both height and total (or actual) body weight (TBW).[2] Several equations

Huang JS, ed. *Curbside Consultation in Pediatric Obesity: 49 Clinical Questions* (pp 185-190).

Table 41-1
Measures of Body Composition

Weight Measure	Equation	Unit	Age Category
BMI	$BMI = \dfrac{TBW\ (kg)}{Height(m)^2}$ Adjust by growth charts for age and sex	Percentile	Child and adolescent
BSA[a]	$BSA = \sqrt{\dfrac{[Height\ (cm) \times TBW\ (kg)]}{3600}}$	m^2	Child and adult
	$BSA = [TBW\ (kg)^{0.5378} \times Height(cm)^{0.3964}] \times 0.024265$	m^2	Infant and child
IBW[b]	$IBW = \dfrac{(Height\ in\ cm)^2\ (1.65)}{1000}$	kg	Child or adolescent 1 to 18 years
	$IBW = 2.396 \times e^{0.01863\ (Height\ in\ cm)}$	kg	Child or adolescent 1 to 17 years
	$IBW = 39kg + 2.27kg$ per inch over 5 feet	kg	Male child ≥5 feet
	$IBW = 42.2kg + 2.27kg$ per inch over 5 feet	kg	Female child ≥5 feet
AdjBW	$AdjBW = IBW(kg) + 0.4[TBW(kg) - IBW(kg)]$		Adult

[a]West nomogram can also be used to determine BSA.

[b]Traub nomogram can also be used to determine IBW for drug dosing. Methods that use growth charts (eg, McLaren and Moore) are used to determine nutritional status.

are available to determine BMI, but they depend on age group (see Table 41-1). Notably, BSA does not account for sex or adipose tissue to lean body weight (LBW).

Originally used by life insurance companies to associate mortality and body size in adults, IBW refers to a body weight that is optimal to maintain a healthy status. The methods to determine IBW in children use the 50th percentile weight for a specific height and/or age (see Table 41-1). A measure similar to IBW is LBW, which is TBW minus the weight of nearly all adipose tissue.

LBW is used interchangeably with fat-free mass, which is the sum of vital organs, extracellular fluid, bones, and muscles. Currently, no method exists to calculate LBW in children.

AdjBW is a measure of body weight between IBW and TBW that incorporates a correction factor in a patient with excess weight. A factor of 0.3 or 0.4 is most commonly used, although values ranging from 0.14 to 0.98 have been suggested. In obese adults, AdjBW has been applied for aminoglycoside and heparin dosing. Minimal literature supports the use of AdjBW for drug dosing in children, although some evidence exists for aminoglycosides using a factor of 0.4.

Pharmacokinetic Alterations

Pediatric drug dosing is generally individualized to the child based on age and body size. Although physiologic maturation that may alter drug pharmacokinetics occurs largely during the neonatal and infant periods, some age-related changes continue into childhood (Table 41-2). Age significantly contributes to drug dosing in neonates, infants, and young children but attenuates in late childhood and adolescence. Age and body size (ie, TBW or BSA) are appropriate measures for normal-sized children; however, using TBW or BSA is inadequate for obese children because the excess weight is not proportionally similar in amounts of lean body and fat mass. Different proportions of both lean body mass and fat mass may alter drug pharmacokinetics and, thereby, dosing.

For systemic drugs, pharmacokinetic alterations are represented by 2 primary parameters that govern dosing: volume of distribution (Vd) and clearance (CL; available via *Physician's Desk Reference*, drug package inserts, Micromedex, Lexicomp). Vd correlates to the total amount of drug disseminated in the body and determines a drug's loading dose. It is largely influenced by the characteristics of the drug itself, as opposed to body composition. For example, a drug's lipophilicity, which is the tendency to concentrate in the lipid tissue, will dictate the extent of drug distribution into adipose tissue and therefore Vd. Some highly lipophilic drugs distribute extensively into adipose tissue, thus increasing Vd, which makes its estimation best by using TBW.[1] However, for drugs that only partially distribute into adipose tissue, AdjBW may be a more conservative measure for Vd. Hydrophilic drugs (eg, aminoglycosides) generally have small Vd and distribute mainly in lean body tissue. IBW (which is closest to LBW) is often used to calculate Vd for hydrophilic drugs, although AdjBW is a reasonable alternative because it accounts for the increase in LBW observed in obese patients.

Adipose tissue carries a small extracellular water volume compared with other tissues (approximately 30% of other body tissue). Obese individuals have decreased total body water per kilogram of actual weight. The effect of this tissue hydration on Vd in obese children is unknown. Plasma protein binding does not appear to change Vd in obese children.

Although Vd establishes the loading dose, CL is needed to estimate maintenance (or chronic) drug dosing. CL accounts for the metabolism and elimination of a drug from the body. Unaffected by a drug's property, CL is regulated by the metabolic capacity and perfusion of certain organs, primarily the liver and kidneys. The liver is the body's primary source for drug metabolism. Obesity during childhood has been associated with an increase in fatty liver, which, in adults, has been shown to impair hepatic blow flow and theoretically drug CL. In addition, obesity in adults has been shown to increase phase 2 reactions (eg, conjugation and glucuronidation) but not phase 1 metabolisms (eg, oxidation, reduction, and hydrolysis). However, CYP3A4, which is responsible for more than 50% of drug metabolism, is reduced in obese patients. As examples, metronidazole, clindamycin, and ketoconazole are metabolized by phase 1 reactions and zidovudine by phase 2 metabolism.

Obese adults have increased creatinine clearance (CrCL), which is a commonly used indicator for renal drug CL. Current methods to estimate CrCL do not accurately predict this increase in

Table 41-2

Age-Related Physiologic Changes That May Alter Drug Pharmacokinetics

Variable	Neonate 0 to 2 months	Infant 3 to 12 months	Child 1 to 12 years	Adolescent < 12 years
Absorption				
Gastric pH	↑(>5)	↑(2 to 4)	↑(2 to 3)	↔
Gastric and intestinal emptying time	↑	↑	↔	↔
Biliary function	↓	↔	↔	↔
Pancreatic function	↓	↔	↔	↔
Gut microbial colonization	↓	↔	↔	↔
Intramuscular absorption	↓	↑	↑ to ↔	↔
Skin permeability and percutaneous absorption	↑	↑	↔	↔
Distribution				
Total body water and extracellular water	↑	↑	↔	↔
Total body fat	↓	↓	Increases by age 5 to 10 years	↔
Total plasma proteins	↓	↓ or ↔	↔	↔
Metabolism				
CYP 1A2	↓	↓	50% by 1 year, ↔ after 1 year	↔
CYP 2C9	30%	↔ by 1 to 6 months	↑(peak 3 to 10 years)	↔ (adult value at puberty)
CYP 2C19	30%	↔ by 6 months	↑(peak 3 to 4 years)	↔ (adult value at puberty)
CYP 2D6	↓(30%)	↔ by 1 year	↔	↔
CYP 2E1	No data	30% to 40%	↔ by 10 years	↔

(continued)

Table 41-2 (continued)
Age-Related Physiologic Changes That May Alter Drug Pharmacokinetics

Variable	Neonate 0 to 2 months	Infant 3 to 12 months	Child 1 to 12 years	Adolescent < 12 years
CYP 3A4	30% to 40%	↔ by 1 year	↑1 to 4 years	↔ at puberty
Uridine 5'-glucuronyl transferase	↓	25% by 3 months	↔ by 6 months to 3 years	↔
N-acetyltransferase 2	↓	↓	↔ past 1 year	↔
Methyltransferase	Up	↔	↔	↔
Sulfotransferase	↓	↑for specific drugs	↑for specific drugs	↔
Renal Elimination				
Glomerular filtration	↓	↔	↔	↔
Tubular secretion and tubular reabsorption	↓	↔	↔	↔

Key: ↔ = same as adult activity; ↓ = decreased activity compared with adults; ↑ = increased activity compared with adults.

obese individuals. Nonetheless, LBW appears to be more accurate than IBW and TBW, which underestimates and overestimates CrCL, respectively. As discussed previously, no method exists to calculate LBW in children currently.

The exact mechanism for the increase in CrCL with obesity is unknown, although animal studies suggest increased kidney mass, increased blood flow to the kidneys, and increased glomerular filtration rate as possibilities. Furthermore, obese adults often suffer from comorbid conditions (eg, hypertension and diabetes) that may compensate for the increase in renal CL. A study of 46 overweight or obese children (BMI ≥85th percentile) matched to 46 controls with normal weight found no significant difference between glomerular filtration rate, serum creatinine, albuminuria, or calciuria. The effect of obesity on renal drug CL in children requires further evaluation.

Because Vd and CL may change with obesity, the elimination half-life (t½) is also likely to vary because it depends on Vd and CL. Exclusively relying on t½ as a measure of drug metabolizing capacity in an obese individual may be misleading (ie, prolonged t½ may originate from a large Vd rather than diminished CL).

The following specific drug examples will illustrate obesity-related alterations in Vd and CL that inevitably affects dosing. Although these examples focus on obesity, incorporating age-related physiologic changes to determine pediatric drug dosing should be underscored. Aminoglycosides are highly hydrophilic antibiotics that distribute mainly into extracellular fluid; therefore, Vd adjusted for TBW is reduced in obese children.[3,4] To achieve an initial therapeutic peak concentration for maximal bactericidal activity, AdjBW rather than IBW is recommended for loading aminoglycosides in obese children. Using TBW may result in peak and trough concentrations that exceed the therapeutic targets and thereby potentially increase the risk for oto- and nephrotoxicity, especially when aminoglycoside CL is unaltered in obese children. Therapeutic drug monitoring is vital to prevent excessive drug concentrations that may lead to toxicities.

Although beta-lactam antibiotics are commonly prescribed in pediatrics, little is known about the effects of obesity on their pharmacokinetics. The Vd and CL, per body weight, of cefazolin appears unaltered in obese children, and TBW has been suggested for its dosing.[3] Unlike beta-lactams, vancomycin is perhaps the most well-studied antimicrobial agent in obese adults. Vancomycin dosing by TBW in obese children has been suggested, although disparity exists because of limiting each dose to 1 gram as many institutions do.[5,6] Nevertheless, adjusting vancomycin dosing based on therapeutic drug monitoring is critical, particularly if TBW is used coupled with evidence suggesting high trough concentrations are associated with increased risk for developing nephrotoxicity.

Daptomycin is similar to vancomycin because TBW is recommended for use in dosing obese adults.[7] Vd adjusted for TBW is similar between normal-weight and obese patients, although using TBW substantially overestimates CrCl in obese population adults. No dosing recommendation is available for pediatric patients aged younger than 18 years, including those who are obese.

Understanding drug properties and physiologic changes that occur with age and obesity is crucial to dosing drugs appropriately in obese children. However, current data are limited, and pharmacokinetic evaluations in obese children are needed to determine optimal drug dosing.

References

1. Kendrick JG, Carr RR, Ensom MH. Pharmacokinetics and drug dosing in obese children. *J Pediatr Pharmacol Ther.* 2010;15(2):94-109.
2. Pai MP. Drug dosing based on weight and body surface area: mathematical assumption and limitations in obese adults. *Pharmacotherapy.* 2012;32(9):856-868.
3. Koshida R, Nakashima E, Taniguchi N, Tsuji A, Benet LZ, Ichimura F. Prediction of the distribution volumes of cefazolin and tobramycin in obese children based on physiological pharmacokinetic concepts. *Pharm Res.* 1989;6(6):486-491.
4. Choi JJ, Moffett BS, McDade EJ, Palazzi DL. Altered gentamicin serum concentration in obese pediatric patients. *Ped Infect Dis J.* 2011;30(4):347-349.
5. Miller M, Miller JL, Hagemann TM, Harrison D, Chavez-Bueno S, Johnson PN. Vancomycin dosage in overweight and obese children. *Am J Health-Syst Pharm.* 2011;68(21):2062-2068.
6. Moffett BS, Kim S, Edwards MS. Vancomycin dosing in obese pediatric patients. *Clin Pediatr (Phila).* 2011;50(5):442-446.
7. Pai MP, Norenberg JP, Anderson T, et al. Influence of morbid obesity on the single-dose pharmacokinetics of daptomycin. *Antimicrob Agents Chemother.* 2007;51(8):2741-2747.

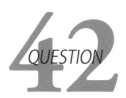

QUESTION

42

WHAT ARE SOME OF THE PARTICULAR RISKS FOR MY OBESE PATIENTS WHO ARE UNDERGOING SURGERY? WHAT STRATEGIES SHOULD BE CONSIDERED TO MINIMIZE THESE RISKS?

Stavra A. Xanthakos, MD, MS

Pediatric obesity, in particular severe obesity, is associated with several comorbid conditions that can increase the risk of anesthetic or surgical complications. The most significant include cardiac abnormalities, obstructive sleep apnea (OSA), type 2 diabetes mellitus, and increased thrombotic risk. These conditions are more often present in severely obese adolescents than in young children but may be undiagnosed prior to surgery. Therefore, a careful preoperative assessment for these factors is important to reduce the risk of anesthetic and surgical complications.

Anesthesia risks can be heightened by obesity because of several additional factors.[1] Visualization of the vocal cords may be more difficult, and intubation may require the aid of a fiber optic bronchoscope. Severely obese patients are more susceptible to perioperative desaturation due to decreased forced vital capacity and functional residual capacity, which can predispose to ventilation/perfusion mismatch and hypoxemia. In addition, pharmacokinetics and pharmacodynamics of anesthetic drugs in obese children are not well understood, and dosages may need to be adjusted based on ideal body weight or estimated lean body mass. Volatile agents accumulate in adipose tissue, which can delay recovery from anesthesia. Postoperatively, opiates for pain control should be dosed on IBW and a further lowering of dosage may be necessary to avoid respiratory depression. Therefore, access to an experienced anesthesia team comfortable with managing obese patients is essential. For severely obese patients, consultation with the anesthesiologist well in advance of surgery is recommended. A history of any prior complications associated with sedation or anesthesia should be elicited during preoperative screening. It is controversial whether metformin use is associated with a greater risk of lactic acidosis. Renal impairment may be a specific risk factor for lactic acidosis associated with metformin use around the time of anesthesia or contrast medium administration for imaging studies. Some imaging guidelines recommend stopping metformin for

Huang JS, ed. *Curbside Consultation in
Pediatric Obesity: 49 Clinical Questions* (pp 191-193).

48 hours prior to and after administration of contrast to patients with known renal impairment. Generally, however, most patients taking metformin can undergo anesthesia safely.

Severe obesity can result in structural alteration in cardiac anatomy (eg, increase in left ventricular mass) and can be associated with acquired long QT syndrome. Diagnosis of prolonged QT interval may require avoidance of certain anesthetics such as sevoflurane, which can induce fatal cardiac arrhythmias in the setting of long QT syndrome. Intraoperative arrest has been reported during bariatric surgery in adults due to long QT syndrome. All adolescents with severe obesity undergoing surgery should be screened with a preoperative electrocardiogram. Hypertension should also be diagnosed and adequately controlled with antihypertensives before surgery.[2]

The presence of OSA in adults undergoing bariatric surgery has been associated with an increased risk of 30-day mortality and thromboembolic risk, but the association with perioperative risks in the adolescent population is unknown.[3] Because OSA is common but often underdiagnosed in severely obese children and adolescents, patients with sleep apnea symptoms, such as snoring and daytime somnolence, should be referred for polysomnography. Continuous pulse oximetry is recommended to monitor patients with OSA pre- and postoperatively. Short-duration anesthetic agents are preferred to enable rapid termination of anesthesia postoperatively. Patients with OSA may also require additional ventilatory support postoperatively. Patients who require continuous positive airway pressure to treat moderate to severe OSA should continue to use it in the immediate postoperative period.

If type 2 diabetes is present, control of blood glucose levels should be optimized preoperatively with a target hemoglobin A1C of < 7% perioperatively.[2] In adolescents undergoing weight loss surgery, blood glucose levels should be monitored closely postoperatively (preprandial and bedtime) because glucose control often rapidly improves in the earliest postoperative days and insulin may need to be adjusted or discontinued to avoid hypoglycemia.

Severely obese patients, including adolescents, are at an increased risk for thromboembolic complications.[2] Therefore, a careful history of any prior thromboembolic complications should be obtained. If any thrombotic history is present in the patient or a first-degree relative, a thrombotic risk evaluation, including laboratory testing for thrombophilic polymorphisms (including factor V Leiden), lipoprotein A levels, and homocysteine levels, should be performed. Consultation with a hematologist is warranted if any positive results emerge. Smoking cessation should be strongly encouraged in adolescent patients and ideally stopped at least 8 weeks preoperatively. In all female adolescents, estrogen-containing oral contraception should be discontinued at least 4 weeks pre- and postoperatively. Progestin-only oral contraceptives may be continued. Limited mobility in the first days postoperatively increases the risk for deep vein thrombosis and pulmonary emboli, which have occurred in severely obese children postoperatively. Therefore, beginning preoperatively and continuing until discharge, low molecular weight heparin is recommended every 12 hours as well as sequential lower-extremity compression devices. Early ambulation is encouraged on the first surgical day whenever feasible. Most thromboembolic complications occur within the first 30 days postoperatively, and patients should be carefully instructed regarding the signs and symptoms to report after discharge.

Adolescents undergoing weight loss surgery can also develop complications requiring more advanced gastrointestinal endoscopic intervention, including balloon dilation of anastomotic strictures, control of bleeding from anastomotic ulcers, and endoluminal stenting of anastomotic leaks. Therefore, availability of an experienced interventional GI endoscopist is necessary.

Finally, to ensure safe care, facilities evaluating and treating severely obese adolescents must be able to accommodate patients whose weights frequently exceed 350 pounds. This includes having access to appropriate beds, chairs, stretchers, commodes, showers/tubs, and imaging and diagnostic equipment suitable for the severely obese patient. In a situation in which weight or girth exceeds the dimension limitations of imaging equipment, for example, alternative methods must be arranged whenever feasible. One example is to perform an upper GI oral contrast study with the patient standing upright rather than lying on a table whose weight limit is often 300 to 350 pounds.[4] Lower-extremity Doppler ultrasonography and pulmonary ventilation/perfusion scanning should be available to evaluate for potential postoperative thromboembolic complications.

Conclusion

Obese children and adolescents are susceptible to several significant comorbid conditions that can increase the risk of perioperative complications. These risks are more prevalent in severely obese children and can be reduced by identifying these factors through preoperative screening and optimizing management prior to and around the time of surgery.

References

1. Baines D. Anaesthetic considerations for the obese child. *Paediatr Respir Rev.* 2011;12(2):144-147.
2. Mechanick JI, Kushner RF, Sugerman HJ, et al. American Association of Clinical Endocrinologists, The Obesity Society, and American Society for Metabolic & Bariatric Surgery Medical Guidelines for Clinical Practice for the perioperative nutritional, metabolic, and nonsurgical support of the bariatric surgery patient. *Surg Obes Relat Dis.* 2008;4(5 Suppl):S109-S184.
3. ASMBS Clinical Issues Committee. Peri-operative management of obstructive sleep apnea. *Surg Obes Relat Dis.* 2012;8(3):e27-e32.
4. Inge TH, Donnelly LF, Vierra M, Cohen AP, Daniels SR, Garcia VF. Managing bariatric patients in a children's hospital: radiologic considerations and limitations. *J Pediatr Surg.* 2005;40(4):609-617.

43 QUESTION

I WANT TO SET UP MY OFFICE TO OPTIMIZE OBESITY SCREENING AND WEIGHT MANAGEMENT. HOW WOULD I SET ABOUT DOING THIS?

Linda L. Hill, MD, MPH

The optimization of obesity care in the pediatric office requires implementing functional office systems. A systematic approach to disease management reduces variability and improves quality of care, productivity, and patient satisfaction.[1] Obesity, although prevalent and easy to identify, is unfortunately often not included in the work up and diagnosis, and even less frequently in the management of clinical issues.[2] Although a number of system-management models exist, I prefer the chronic care model (CCM) as a clear and evidenced-based model for weight management (Figure 43-1).[3,4] The CCM includes the following components particularly relevant to obesity care: delivery system design, decision support, and clinical information systems in the office, as well as community resources. Integration of these components into your practice will optimize obesity screening and weight management. The goal is to have a prepared team ready for interaction with an informed and activated patient. You can move toward achieving that goal with the following steps.

Starting with your office, look at your delivery system. You need adequate staff to manage the components of obesity interventions, such as screening, counseling, and follow-up (Table 43-1). The team members can be cross-trained or have their individual areas of expertise, depending on the size of your office. Begin with screening, checking that each visit includes the accurate measurement of height and weight and the calculation of body mass index (BMI) and BMI/weight/height percentiles. Where appropriate, incorporate the completion of assessment forms into pre-visit activities, such as the Health & Obesity: Prevention and Education SHAPES Assessment form (Figure 43-2).[5]

Your office should provide the types of visits needed to manage obesity. If you have decided that including individual visits, group visits, and nutrition counseling are all appropriate for obesity management in your practice, design these visits in detail, identifying the team members and

Huang JS, ed. *Curbside Consultation in Pediatric Obesity: 49 Clinical Questions* (pp 195-199).
© 2014 Taylor & Francis Group

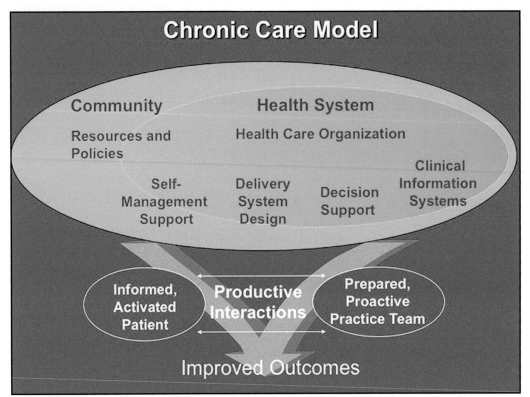

Figure 43-1. The CCM provides the system components for effective office management of obesity and other chronic diseases. (Reprinted with permission from Wagner EH. Chronic disease management: what will it take to improve care for chronic illness? *Eff Clin Pract.* 1998;1(1):2-4.)

expertise requirements for implementation. I have found group visits useful for chronic disease management, including obesity, and would encourage you to strongly consider incorporating them into your practice. Plan and write out the components of each activity: who will conduct the intervention, what the intervention will include, when the intervention will be offered, and additional support staff or equipment needed.

The decision support component of the CCM includes the development of protocols and guidelines for your practice and the appropriate training. Your team needs to be trained on evidence-based management of obesity and how to address barriers to action.[6,7] In-office seminars, online seminars, or conferences can enhance their expertise. Where possible, incorporate automated calculations and determination of BMI percentiles into your system; these generally can be performed with electronic health records. If using paper charts, provide BMI calculators and appropriate graphs for the staff who obtain the vital signs. Include obesity management in your quality improvement program. Audit your obesity care as part of general quality improvement activities.[1] The quality improvement components should include defining the steps to optimization of practice, measuring the achievement, providing feedback, and making appropriate changes to the practice based on the audit results. Ongoing staff training ensures maintenance of competency and brings new team members up to date. Staff turnover is inevitable, so have periodic training in place.

Your patients should also be trained on the ability to make informed decisions. Obesity self-management is a crucial component of obesity control, and training parents as well as patients is needed. Appropriate information, including materials, references, and websites, will improve

Table 43-1
Office Setup Components

Component	*Tasks/Items*	*Staffing Options*
Delivery system	Screening: height, weight, BMI calculation, assessment forms	Medical assistants, nursing
	Individual visits, group visits, nutrition counseling	Physicians, psychologist, health educators, nutritionists
Professional decision support	Staff training	Physicians, online training, CME courses
	Electronic health records	IT staff
	Quality improvement	QI staff: Physicians, nursing
Patient decision support	Materials, references, websites	IT staff, health educators
	Group visits	Physicians, psychologist, health educators, nutritionists
Clinical information systems	Registries, follow-up	Nursing, case managers
Community resources	Schools	Physicians, nurses, managers
	Recreation facilities	
	Park access	
Office resources	Furniture	Managers
	Scales	
	Health messages	

Abbreviations: CME, continuing medical education; IT, information technology.

their decision processes and should be included in individual and group counseling. Numerous technological devices are available, such as smartphone applications, pedometers, accelerometers, and Web-based systems. I have found it helpful to become familiar with 1 to 2 examples in each category to help patients choose devices that work with their lifestyle and level of technological expertise.

The clinical information systems component includes tracking and follow-up of patients. You should enter your patients with obesity into a registry. The follow-up should not be left to chance; your obese patients should be enrolled and tracked, with case managers (either designated individuals or cross-trained staff) following up on appointments, referrals, and progress. You may

HOPE SHAPES Lifestyle Questionnaire

This form will help your health care provider understand your lifestyle. Please respond to each item by yourself or with the help of your parent. Also, indicate if you are willing to talk to your health care provider about improving in each specific area.

Patient Name_____

Date of Birth_____

S **SODA** LIMIT SODA & SWEETENED BEVERAGES	How many ounces of sodas or sweetened beverages or fruit juices do you (your child) drink each day?	_____ oz/day
	Are you willing to work on this area?	☐ Yes ☐ No
H **EAT MEALS AT HOME** LIMIT EATING OUT AT RESTAURANTS	How many meals do you (your child) eat at home each week?	_____ meals/wk
	Are you willing to work on this area?	☐ Yes ☐ No
A **BE ACTIVE** BE ACTIVE DAILY FOR AT LEAST 1 HOUR	How many days each week do you (your child) play outside or exercise for at least 60 minutes?	_____ days/wk
	Are you willing to work on this area?	☐ Yes ☐ No
P **PORTION CONTROL** WATCH YOUR PORTIONS AT EVERY MEAL	How often do you (your child) take second helpings? (Mark one)	☐ Almost Never ☐ Not Often ☐ Sometimes ☐ Often ☐ Always
	Are you willing to work on this area?	☐ Yes ☐ No
E **EAT BREAKFAST** EAT BREAKFAST EVERY MORNING	How many days a week do you (your child) eat breakfast?	_____ days/wk
	Are you willing to work on this area?	☐ Yes ☐ No
S **SCREEN TIME** REDUCE TV, VIDEO GAME PLAY & COMPUTER TIME TO 2 HOURS PER DAY	How many hours each day do you/your child spend watching TV or playing video/computer games? (do not include computer use for homework)	_____ hrs/day
	Are you willing to work on this area?	☐ Yes ☐ No

Figure 43-2. The Health & Obesity: Prevention and Education SHAPES Assessment form.

already be doing this with other chronic diseases (eg, diabetes, asthma). These registries will aid in the assessment of your progress on obesity management because you will be able to query the system for trends in BMI among at-risk patients. Follow-up calls go beyond reminder and recall of appointments and can be used to enforce behavioral interventions, provide patients and their parents with technical support, and aid in reinforcing positive behaviors.

The community is an important component of effective pediatric obesity management. I like to be well acquainted with the communities where my patients are living so I am aware of their access to appropriate community resources, such as healthy food, safe parks, walkable neighborhoods, and recreation facilities. It is important to be aware of the resources in your community (or lack thereof) because advocacy for improvement can be as important a component of obesity management as the in-office changes. Include the schools in your assessments because your patients' diet and exercise are strongly influenced by the options there (see Question 49).

On a more practical note, design your office to accommodate your overweight patients (and their parents). For individual counseling and group classes, for example, check the weight limits and width of your chairs, including the waiting room. Make sure your scale supports at least 500 pounds, especially if you treat adolescents. Gown and exam tables should also be adequately sized. Provide confidentiality for weight measures. Design your waiting room to deliver positive health messages and reading/video materials (see Question 40).

The resources needed to provide adequate office screening and management of obesity, including personnel, equipment, electronic health record support, and administration time, require support from the health system leadership. Your role as a pediatrician includes community advocacy and the education of administrative leaders in your system on the importance of this major public health problem.

References

1. Barlow S, Dietz W. Management of child and adolescent obesity: summary and recommendations based on reports from pediatricians, pediatric nurse practitioners, and registered dietitians. *Pediatrics.* 2002;110(1 Pt 2):236-238.
2. O'Brien SH, Holubkov R, Reis EC. Identification, evaluation, and management of obesity in an academic primary care center. *Pediatrics.* 2004;114(2):e154-e159.
3. Wagner EH. Chronic disease management: what will it take to improve care for chronic illness? *Eff Clin Pract.* 1998;1(1):2-4.
4. Coleman K, Austin BT, Brach C, Wagner EH. Evidence on the Chronic Care Model in the new millennium. *Health Aff (Millwood).* 2009;28(1):75-85.
5. Huang J, Pokala P, Hill L, et al. The Health and Obesity: Prevention and Education (HOPE) Curriculum project—curriculum development. *Pediatrics.* 2009;124(5):1438-1446.
6. Story MT, Neumark-Stzainer DR, Sherwood NE, et al. Management of child and adolescent obesity: attitudes, barriers, skills, and training needs among health care professionals. *Pediatrics.* 2002;110(1 Pt 2):210-214.
7. Edmunds L, Waters E, Elliott E. Evidence based paediatrics: evidence based management of childhood obesity. *BMJ.* 2001;323(7318):916-919.

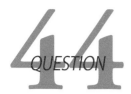

How Does Treatment of Obesity Differ According to Age?

Stephanie Knatz, PhD and Kerri N. Boutelle, PhD

Primary treatments for pediatric obesity include behavioral management strategies and lifestyle interventions aimed at achieving a negative energy balance. Behavioral family-based treatment (FBT) for pediatric obesity is currently the most effective treatment for children of all ages, including preschool-aged children, school-aged children, and adolescents. FBT targets the most influential factors associated with weight, namely diet, physical activity, and sedentary activity by using behavioral strategies that are known to be effective in increasing behaviors that lead to weight loss (eg, physical activity, fruit and vegetable consumption, decreased calories) and reducing behaviors that lead to weight gain (eg, screen time, consumption of high-fat foods).[1] This method has been shown to be most effective in reducing weight when parents are involved.[2] For children of all ages, parental involvement is a critical factor for achieving weight loss but must be tailored to be developmentally appropriate for the child. Thus, despite the age of the child, treatment should focus on increasing healthy behaviors and reducing unhealthy behaviors associated with weight management and include parental and/or caretaker involvement and support. Although there is little formal distinction of FBT for children of different ages, some important developmental considerations should be taken into account to tailor treatment to the child and his or her family.[3] These include autonomy levels, motivation, peer influence, and self-regulatory ability.

In addition, the weight of the child should also be considered because some children may be able to reduce their body mass index by growing into their weight and maintaining a stable weight.[1] It is important to consider how treatment should be modified to take into account developmental abilities while still focusing on the factors known to be critical for success in pediatric weight loss.

Huang JS, ed *Curbside Consultation in
Pediatric Obesity: 49 Clinical Questions* (pp 201-204).
© 2014 Taylor & Francis Group

Preschool-Aged Children

It is important to intervene with children during their preschool years because it is the time of the life during which eating behaviors are beginning to form into habits that can often endure through adulthood. With children this young, parents are responsible for making changes in diet and activity levels. Direct intervention with the child is not necessary. Instructing parents on appropriate ways to intervene at this early age (ages 0 to 4 years) provides the opportunity to introduce healthy behaviors that will lead to reduced risk of overweight and obesity at later life stages.

Providers should focus on parental competencies in the arena of diet and physical activity. Because eating behaviors and taste preferences are being formed during this developmental period, interventions should focus on the development of preference for healthy foods and the reduction of high-calorie foods. Children's taste preferences can be influenced by exposure to foods, with more exposures being associated with increased liking. Accordingly, parents should be instructed to increase exposure to healthy foods, including a variety of fruits and vegetables, while decreasing exposure to foods that are high in calories. During this developmental period, children may be more or less willing to try new foods, but parents should continue to emphasize and offer fruits and vegetables at every meal and snack. At these young ages, children are also less influenced by external cues to regulate eating behaviors and better attuned to hunger and satiety. Although these signals might not be completely intact in an obese preschooler, parents should be aware of their own feeding practices, including permissive feeding (ie, letting the child have whatever he or she asks for), restrictive feeding (ie, making foods off-limits), or exerting pressure to eat (ie, finish your plate). Parents' assistance in improving their child's diet should be focused mainly around increasing the variety and exposure of healthy foods, such as fruits and vegetables, while reducing exposure and variety to unhealthy, high-calorie foods and making healthy foods more appealing.

With regard to physical activity, parents are responsible for ensuring that physical activity is integrated into their children's routines. The best way to do this is to incorporate activity into everyday life, such as daily visits to the park or playtime outside. Because young children can become bored and/or tired easily, physical activity can be broken into small increments throughout the day. At this age, involvement with play and enjoyment of physical activity should be the focus rather than organized team play or physical activity as a requirement. Parents of children younger than age 2 years should be discouraged from allowing screen time because of the potential negative effects associated with both foreground and background screen time for children in this age range. Screen time should be limited to 2 hours per day for children aged 2 to 4 years.[4] Turning off screens may be enough to encourage preschoolers to be more active.

Sleep is another important consideration for children of this age because of the associations between lack of sleep and weight gain.[5] Providers should review appropriate sleep guidelines with parents and ensure that children are getting an appropriate amount of sleep (see Question 8).

School-Aged Children

As children transition into this age range (4 to 12 years), there is typically increased exposure to outside eating environments that often include high-calorie foods (eg, birthday parties, school, friends' houses). It is important that parents focus on maintaining the quality of children's diet throughout this time and attempt to limit the consumption of high-calorie foods that become more popular to consume during this age, such as soda and other sugar-sweetened beverages. Dietary interventions during this age range should focus on increasing the consumption of fruits and vegetables and reducing the consumption of foods that are high in fat and sugar. At this age, children are capable of learning about healthy choices, and parents should attempt to involve their children in reading nutrition labels and understanding the role of healthy eating. However, because children at this age have a limited capacity to make healthy choices and practice self-control in the face of temptation (eg, not eat the brownie on their plate), parents should be coached on the importance of controlling the home food environment to reduce exposure and temptations for unhealthy foods. Parents are still primarily responsible for the majority of children's food choices at this stage and thus should be responsible for setting a meal structure and assisting children in making healthy choices. Specifically, parents should encourage a healthy breakfast and provide family meals, both of which have been associated with better weight outcomes.

Sedentary activity can also increase during these years, so parents should focus efforts on limited screen time and continue to facilitate physical activity. Activity recommendations for children include 90 minutes of physical activity and less than 2 hours of screen time per day. Physical activity goals can be met by incorporating healthy family activities that involve the entire family and encourage children to be more active. In addition, parents should consider introducing structured activity such as team sports or other organized physical activity. After-school activities and team sports are excellent ways to ensure that children meet their physical activity requirements on a regular basis.

Children at this age are also highly responsive to praise and positive reinforcement from their parents. Parents should be instructed to focus on praising behaviors that are associated with improving weight (eg, "I noticed that you chose an apple for your snack today instead of chips; I am so proud of you for making a healthy choice!"). Since children in this age range are not always internally motivated, parents can use a positive reinforcement system, by which kids earn points toward rewards for engaging in healthy behaviors associated with weight loss (eg, child earns 1 point daily for doing at least 30 minutes of physical activity) that can be traded in for a reward.

Adolescents

Adolescence marks a shift toward increased autonomy and independence and greater peer influence. Although adolescents both desire and require more independence, studies have shown that parental involvement in treatment results in better outcomes.[6] Parental involvement in weight loss treatment changes as their teenagers spend more time with their peers and have increased ability to make choices about food and activity levels independently. The parental role during this stage becomes more collaborative, and parents need to be on the same team as their teenager. Conversations regarding health outcomes and teenagers' goals might be useful to allow parents and teens to have common measurable goals to work toward. In addition, one of the most important and effective ways for parents to be involved in their teenager's weight loss is by modeling healthy behaviors and participating in recommended lifestyle changes with their teens. If teens are lacking in motivation, parents can consider implementing a motivator system similar to the one described earlier that has teens earn points for engaging in healthy behaviors. The rewards for this motivator program need to be tailored to the teenager's developmental level and interests.

Adolescent obesity is associated with decreased self-esteem, peer victimization, and other psychopathology. These issues become more prevalent during adolescence in general; however, obese teenagers are more likely to experience these issues as a result of their weight status. It is important to assess for the presence of these mental health issues and, if necessary, ensure that teenagers are getting the appropriate treatment.

Conclusion

Similar principles of decreasing caloric intake through the removal of high-calorie foods, increasing physical activity (both planned and lifestyle activity) and decreased screen time are key components to FBT and to parents assisting their child in weight loss. Parental involvement is key for all children and most adolescents, although parental involvement and influence varies as children develop.

References

1. Barlow SE, Dietz WH. Obesity evaluation and treatment: expert committee recommendations. The Maternal and Child Health Bureau, Health Resources and Services Administration and the Department of Health and Human Services. *Pediatrics.* 1998;102(3):E29.
2. Golan M, Weizman A, Apter A, Fainaru M. Parents as the exclusive agents of change in the treatment of childhood obesity. *Am J Clin Nutr.* 1998;67(6):1130-1135.
3. Jelalian E, Steele RG, eds. *Handbook of Child and Adolescent Obesity.* New York, NY: Springer; 2008.
4. Council on Communications and Media, Brown A. Media use by children younger than 2 years. *Pediatrics.* 2011;128(5):1040-1045.
5. Chen X, Beydoun MA, Wang Y. Is sleep duration associated with childhood obesity? A systematic review and meta-analysis. *Obesity (Silver Spring).* 2012;16(2):265-274.
6. Jelalian E, Hart CN, Mehlenbeck RS, et al. Predictors of attrition and weight loss in an adolescent weight control program. *Obesity (Silver Spring).* 2012;16(6):1318-1323.

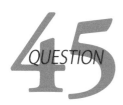

WHAT ARE THE SPECIAL CHALLENGES OF MANAGING OBESITY IN THE CHILD WITH AUTISM?

Colleen Taylor Lukens, PhD

Autism spectrum disorders are a class of developmental disorders characterized by impairments in social interaction and communication, stereotyped behaviors, and developmental delays. Studies suggest similar or even higher rates of obesity in children with autism than in the general population, and this prevalence may be related to maladaptive dietary patterns, minimal engagement in physical activity, limited responsiveness to typical intervention strategies, and medication management of behavioral difficulties.[1] However, once these contributing factors are identified, treatment approaches can be effectively altered and medication regimens adjusted to meet the unique needs of children with autism and other developmental disabilities.

Factors Contributing to Obesity in Children With Autism

Diets rich in calories and fat and poor in nutrient-dense foods are significant contributors to obesity, and this dietary composition can be a result of selective eating behavior. Selective eating is a common problem of early childhood, resulting from a combination of factors including diminishing appetite, the presence of neophobia (mild fear of new things), and the increasing desire for independence from caregivers. In typically developing children, these issues most often resolve in the preschool years; however, in children with autism, food selectivity often persists into school age and adolescence.[2] Characteristics associated with a diagnosis of autism can exacerbate food selectivity, subsequently leading to inadequate nutrient intake.[3,4] For example, children with autism may demonstrate severe food refusal behavior that is physically difficult to manage, increasing the likelihood that a parent will remove food that has been refused and offer highly preferred foods. As well, limited responsiveness

Huang JS, ed. *Curbside Consultation in Pediatric Obesity: 49 Clinical Questions* (pp 205-208).
© 2014 Taylor & Francis Group

to social cues may decrease the effectiveness of peer and parental modeling of healthy eating habits in altering a child's mealtime behavior. Finally, children with autism present with a characteristic preference for routine and sameness, which may contribute to restricted dietary preferences.

Just as in the population of typically developing children, obesity in children with autism is also related to limited physical activity and increased sedentary behavior. Motor impairments that have been identified at higher rates in children with autism (eg, hypotonia, motor apraxia, global deficits in gross motor skills) may preclude involvement in or further decrease a child's motivation to participate in physical activity.[5] Impairments in communication also adversely impact the ability of a child with autism to engage in physical activity. As well, atypical and repetitive behavior may lead to alienation from peers, preventing participation in group physical activity. Children with autism may withdraw from physical activities that have a social element and subsequently participate in more isolating and sedentary activity.

Finally, medication management of severe behavioral difficulties in children with autism can contribute to obesity. Medications commonly prescribed to reduce severely disruptive and self-injurious behavior in children with autism (eg, antipsychotic medications) are associated with rapid and excessive weight gain. When paired with poor nutrition and inadequate physical activity as described previously, weight management becomes more difficult with increasingly adverse implications for physical health.

Intervention

A core component of obesity intervention is increasing positive health behavior related to diet and exercise. Common elements of such intervention include education regarding nutrition and physical activity, monitoring of food and caloric intake, increasing daily physical activity, and altering components of diet to optimize nutritional intake. The same characteristics that are thought to contribute to selective eating and limited physical activity in children with autism also adversely affect the effectiveness of these intervention and weight management strategies.

Typical interventions can be altered to effectively manage obesity in children with developmental disabilities. For example, although an individual with autism may not be responsive to nutrition education or may not be able to self-monitor diet and exercise routines because of cognitive difficulties, these components of intervention can be effectively taught to primary caregivers. As well, the characteristic preference for routine seen in children with autism is often a significant obstacle to altering diet and exercise regimens. However, capitalizing on this preference by gradually and clearly establishing new routines and rules around food and physical activity can be beneficial when working with the child with autism. As well, tailoring incentive programs to the child with autism can optimize participation in making these lifestyle changes.

Adapting medication regimens in children with autism is also critical when intervening around weight management. It is important for physicians to carefully examine costs and benefits, both long and short term, of using medications associated with rapid weight gain. This is an important area for intervention in the primary care setting because physicians can carefully monitor weight gain when such medications are introduced and consider alternative interventions around disruptive behavior if weight gain becomes excessive. Finally, referral to a child and adolescent psychiatrist can be beneficial in optimizing medication regimens in children with autism.

Role of the Primary Care Physician

Identifying specific obstacles to effective weight management is an important first step to intervention and can facilitate appropriate referral if necessary. For example, if a parent demonstrates

---

Table 45-1
Areas for Assessment

Selective Eating
- How often does the caregiver offer new foods?
- How severe is the child's food refusal behavior?
- How does the caregiver respond to food refusal behavior?
- How responsive is the child to modeling of healthy eating habits?
- How strong is the child's preference for routine?

Limited Physical Activity
- Are motor impairments or deficits in gross motor skills present?
- What is the child's level of interest in group physical activity?
- Does the child demonstrate a preference for sedentary activity?
- How often does the caregiver attempt to engage the child in physical activity?
- How does the caregiver respond if the child refuses to engage in physical activity?

---

limited knowledge regarding the composition of an age-typical diet, nutritional counseling would be the recommended first step. However, if a caregiver reports difficulty with establishing clear expectations and setting limits around food preferences and sedentary activities because of resultant disruptive behavior, consultation with a behavioral specialist would be more appropriate.

Asking specific questions about a child's behavior and caregiver responses during mealtimes and around physical activity can yield helpful information about these obstacles (Table 45-1). For example:

- "How does your child respond if you put a new food on his plate?"
- "How do you respond if your child gets upset at mealtimes?"
- "How does your child respond if you ask her to go for a walk?"
- "How do you respond if your child refuses to go for a walk?"

Caregiver responses to these questions may also suggest some plausible first steps (Table 45-2), keeping in mind that overall, children with autism benefit from treatment packages that incorporate high levels of support and supervision, establish clear and manageable goals, and embrace gradual and systematic change. For example, a primary care physician can provide anticipatory guidance to caregivers regarding the establishment of a consistent mealtime and physical activity schedule and routine. A visual schedule (sequential pictorial presentation of a series of tasks) is one such strategy for providing clear expectations and establishing a new daily routine. Also, pediatricians can encourage a caregiver to expose a child to new foods through participation in meal preparation or placement of new foods close to a child's plate at mealtimes without expectation to eat. Finally, gradual approaches to altering dietary variety can be recommended, such as offering baked rather than fried versions of preferred foods or decreasing portion sizes of high-calorie foods one piece at a time.

Alternatively, caregiver responses can reveal information regarding parent-child interaction or behavior management difficulties that limit the effectiveness of such basic strategies. In such

Table 45-2
Primary Care Practice

- Teach caregivers to provide high levels of support and supervision
- Establish clear and manageable goals
- Establish regular schedules and routines around mealtime and physical activity
- Provide exposure to nonpreferred foods via engagement in meal preparation activity
- Encourage visual and tactile exploration of new foods with limited expectation to eat
- Encourage gradual changes in diet/exercise routines using an incremental approach
- Encourage the family to engage in repeated practice
- Consult with dietitians, educational professionals, and behavioral specialists
- Adjust medication regimens to include those less commonly associated with weight gain

instances, coordinating care with a child's behavioral health clinicians or educational personnel, including teachers, occupational therapists, and physical therapists, may be beneficial.

Conclusion

It is important for primary care practitioners to be aware of the unique challenges faced when managing obesity in children with autism. The development of food selectivity and limitations on physical activity along with use of medications associated with rapid weight gain are likely contributors to higher rates of obesity in children with autism than in typically developing children. Characteristics associated with a diagnosis of an autism spectrum disorder can also adversely affect the effectiveness of intervention strategies. Identifying obstacles to effective weight management, supporting gradual and systematic change, and engaging in care coordination with educational and behavioral health clinicians is crucial to the success of any weight management intervention for children with autism.

References

1. Curtin C, Anderson SE, Must A, Bandini L. The prevalence of obesity in children with autism: a secondary data analysis using nationally representative data from the National Survey of Children's Health. *BMC Pediatr.* 2010;10:11.
2. Williams KE, Foxx RM. *Treating Eating Problems of Children With Autism Spectrum Disorders and Developmental Disabilities: Interventions for Professionals and Parents.* Dallas, TX: Pro-Ed; 2007.
3. Schreck KA, Williams K. Food preferences and factors influencing food selectivity for children with autism spectrum disorders. *Res Dev Disabil.* 2006;27(4):353-363.
4. Bandini LG, Anderson SE, Curtin C, et al. Food selectivity in children with autism spectrum disorders and typically developing children. *J Pediatr.* 2010;157(2):259-264.
5. Matson ML, Matson JL, Beighley JS. Comorbidity of physical and motor problems in children with autism. *Res Dev Disabil.* 2011;32(6):2304-2308.

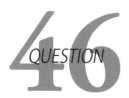

WHAT DRUGS ARE AVAILABLE TO TREAT OBESITY IN CHILDREN?

Kirsten La, PharmD, BCPS and
Jennifer Le, PharmD, MAS, BCPS-ID, FCCP, FCSHP

The Expert Committee on childhood obesity, composed of 15 national health care organizations formed by the American Medical Association in collaboration with the Health Resources and Service Administration and the Centers for Disease Control, recommends the use of drugs only after lifestyle modifications fail to meet weight reduction goals or improve significant comorbidities, which may include diabetes mellitus, dyslipidemias, metabolic syndrome, nonalcoholic fatty liver disease, gallstone disease, and pseudotumor cerebri.[1,2] A 4-stage, stepwise approach is proposed to treat child and adolescent overweight and obesity after a diagnosis based on age- and sex-specific growth curves of body mass index (BMI; see Question 2 regarding BMI definitions). Each step progresses in treatment intensity, and the decision to advance to later stages depends on individual patient goals and response. Variations on dietary modification, physical activity, and behavioral therapy form the first 3 stages. Pharmacotherapy, very low-calorie diet, and weight control surgery are possible treatment options in stage 4 when lifestyle interventions prove ineffective. Although no definitive recommendations are available for duration of drug use, the Expert Committee advocates pharmacotherapy for children aged 11 years and older who meet both of the following criteria:

- Failed stages 1 to 3 interventions, *and*

- Have a BMI > 99th percentile, or a BMI > 95th percentile with significant comorbidities[1]

When considering pharmacotherapy, children should be referred to experts with experience in using anti-obesity medications in youth. Referral to pediatric weight management centers operating under a protocol by multidisciplinary teams is also recommended.[1] The long-term adverse effects of medications used to treat childhood obesity are unknown. Furthermore, the weight reduction effects of these drugs are generally modest and plateau within 4 to 6 months of treatment. There may also be concerns of weight regain when medications are stopped.[2]

Huang JS, ed. *Curbside Consultation in
Pediatric Obesity: 49 Clinical Questions* (pp 209-212).
© 2014 Taylor & Francis Group

Table 46-1

Medications for Weight Control[3]

Drug Name	Pediatric Dose	Adverse Effects
Orlistat	120 mg 3 times a day before meals	Abdominal pain, oily spotting, flatus with discharge, oily/fatty stool, fecal urgency and increased defecation
Metformin	500 to 1000 mg twice daily	Nausea, vomiting, diarrhea, flatulence, and lactic acidosis (less common but more serious)

There are 3 primary mechanisms of action for pharmacotherapies used to treat obesity: increase the concentration or inhibit the reuptake of neurotransmitters (eg, norepinephrine, serotonin, and dopamine, which suppress appetite), inhibit the uptake of nutrients such as fats, or activate receptors that suppress appetite or affect metabolism. Among the 5 Food and Drug Administration (FDA)-approved medications, phentermine (Adipex-P, Suprenza), phentermine-topiramate (Qsymia), and lorcaserin (Belviq) serve as anorexiants and are approved for use only in adults. Phentermine, phentermine-topiramate, and lorcaserin are scheduled IV controlled substances. Diethylpropion (Tenuate) is another scheduled IV controlled anorectic substance that is approved for adolescents aged older than 16 years; however, efficacy data are limited in the pediatric population, and it is not mentioned as a treatment option in pediatric obesity recommendations.[1,2] Other appetite suppressants, including sibutramine, are no longer available in the United States, primarily for their adverse effect profiles. Specifically, sibutramine was withdrawn in 2010 when the Sibutramine Cardiovascular Outcomes Trial uncovered an increased risk of cardiovascular events with its use.

Compared with other drugs used in the treatment of obesity, orlistat uniquely decreases systemic fat absorption by reversibly inhibiting gastrointestinal (GI) lipase. At the recommended doses, approximately 30% of dietary fat absorption is inhibited by orlistat (Table 46-1). It is available as prescription (Xenical) and over-the-counter formulations (Alli). Only the prescription formulation is approved for children aged 12 years and older. Pharmacokinetic studies show that orlistat is minimally absorbed. As such, the most common adverse effects are mild and transient GI effects. These adverse effects may increase with ingestion of high-fat meals; therefore, high-fat meals should be avoided. Since orlistat inhibits the absorption of fat-soluble vitamins (ie, A, D, E, and K), a multivitamin should be supplemented daily during the course of therapy. Orlistat is contraindicated in patients with chronic malabsorption syndrome and cholestasis.[3,4]

The efficacy and safety of orlistat was evaluated in a 1-year, randomized, double-blind, placebo-controlled, multicenter study by Chanoin et al.[5] The ages of subjects ($N=539$) ranged from 12 to 16 years; all subjects had a BMI at least 2 units above the 95th percentile; and 25% of subjects had metabolic syndrome. In conjunction with diet, exercise, and behavioral therapy for both study groups, the reduction in BMI was significantly higher with orlistat compared with placebo (-0.55 vs +0.31 kg/m^2; *P* = 0.001). At least twice as many subjects treated with orlistat compared with placebo had a 5% and 10% BMI reduction (27% and 13% vs 16% and 5%, respectively).[5] Response at 12 weeks correlated with overall weight loss at the end of the 1-year treatment.[3] Other studies, which are not as well designed and are limited by much smaller sample sizes, have reported mixed results. When comparing orlistat with placebo or control, some studies showed a significant change in BMI with orlistat, up to -4.2 kg/m^2, whereas others have not.[4] In regard to cardiovascular and metabolic measures, the Chanoine et al[5] study found that the orlistat group showed significant decreases in waist and hip circumference as well as diastolic blood pressure compared with placebo. No significant decreases in lipid, insulin, and glucose biomarkers were observed.[5]

Other medications, such as metformin, have been studied in children but are not FDA approved specifically for treating obesity. Metformin is indicated for the treatment of type 2 diabetes mellitus in children aged 10 years and older, and is being increasingly studied as a possible medication for weight reduction in children (see Table 46-1).[3] Metformin is a biguanide antihyperglycemic agent that promotes weight loss by modulating metabolism. Its multiple mechanisms of action for controlling diabetes mellitus are inhibition of intestinal glucose absorption, decrease in hepatic glucose production, and increase in peripheral insulin sensitivity. Although the common adverse effects of metformin are confined to GI symptoms, serious events, such as lactic acidosis, can occur, particularly in patients with decreased renal clearance or hypoxemia and those taking alcohol concurrently with metformin. Metformin is contraindicated in patients with renal disease or dysfunction. Drug discontinuation is recommended for those with liver dysfunction or receiving IV contrast agents.[6]

Three randomized, double-blind, placebo-controlled trials of children aged 9 years and older lasting 6 months showed discrepant results in BMI change. One study of 120 subjects showed a significant reduction in BMI with metformin (28.5 to 26.7 kg/m^2; *P* < 0.001) and no significant change with placebo.[4,6] Two other studies with 85 and 70 subjects showed no significant change in BMI compared to placebo. Results were also conflicting for improvements in biomarkers of insulin resistance or glucose metabolism.[6]

Many studies evaluating metformin against placebo included children aged 9 years and older and lasted for 6 months or less.[6] However, a randomized, double-blind, placebo-controlled trial included subjects as young as age 6 years (range, 6 to 12 years). In this study, 100 obese, insulin-resistant children received either metformin or placebo for 6 months. Compared with placebo, metformin treatment resulted in significantly less weight gain at 6 months (+1.47 vs +4.85 kg; *P* < 0.001). In a randomized, double-blind, placebo-controlled trial of 77 subjects aged 13 years and older, a significant change in mean BMI compared with the placebo arm was observed at 48 weeks (-0.9 vs +0.2 kg/m^2; *P* = 0.03). This is notably the longest study to date.[3]

Overall, the clinical trials evaluating metformin for weight loss in obese pediatric patients are limited by small sample sizes and short durations. These studies also varied in study population, with some targeting children and adolescents exhibiting hyperinsulinemia or impaired glucose tolerance. With these limitations and variations, more robust studies of metformin for use in children to control weight are warranted since preliminary findings are promising. Other medications with non-obesity indications may be useful in decreasing or maintaining weight but have not been studied for the treatment of childhood obesity (Table 46-2).

Orlistat and potentially metformin are 2 viable options for treating obesity in pediatric patients who are unresponsive to lifestyle management and have significant comorbidities. The effects of these pharmacotherapies are modest at best and are often studied in conjunction with lifestyle modifications. Furthermore, the therapeutic and safety effects beyond 1 year of therapy remain unknown because long-term controlled studies are limited. Although medications may provide short-term benefits, frequent weight regain following discontinuation of therapy may limit their

Table 46-2

Medications That May Lead to Weight Loss[3]

Drug Name	Approved Indications	Proposed Mechanism of Action
Topiramate	Anticonvulsant	Appetite suppressant
Bupropion	Antidepressant	Appetite suppressant
Fluoxetine	Antidepressant	Appetite suppressant
Octreotide	Somatostatin analogue	Decrease insulin resistance

usefulness. Lifestyle interventions remain the mainstay of therapy for long-term management of childhood obesity. As such, medication use should be considered with lifestyle modifications only when lifestyle interventions fail to meet goals and should be prescribed by clinicians with experience in use of such agents in the pediatric population.

References

1. Barlow SE; Expert Committee. Expert Committee recommendations regarding the prevention, assessment and treatment of child and adolescent overweight and obesity: summary report. *Pediatrics*. 2007;120(Suppl 4):S164-S192.
2. August GP, Caprio S, Fennoy I. Prevention and treatment of pediatric obesity: an Endocrine Society clinical practice guideline based on expert opinion. *J Clin Endocrinol Metab*. 2008;93(12):4576-4599.
3. Sherafat-Kazemzadeh R, Yanovski SZ, Yanovski JA. Pharmacotherapy for childhood obesity: present and future prospects. *Int J Obes (Lond)*. 2013;37(1):1-15.
4. Rogovik AL, Chanoine JP, Goldman RD. Pharmacotherapy and weight-loss supplements for treatment of paediatric obesity. *Drugs*. 2010;12:70(3):335-346.
5. Chanoine JP, Hampl S, Jensen C. Effect of orlistat on weight and body composition in obese adolescents: a randomized, controlled trial. *JAMA*. 2005;293(23):2873-2883.
6. Brufani C, Fintini D, Nobili V, Patera PI, Cappa M, Brufani M. Use of metformin in pediatric age. *Pediatr Diabetes*. 2011;12(6):580-588.

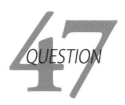

THERE ARE A NUMBER OF COMMERCIAL WEIGHT LOSS PROGRAMS. WHICH ARE SAFE, EFFECTIVE, AND APPROPRIATE TO RECOMMEND TO OBESE OR OVERWEIGHT CHILDREN?

Rohit Gupta, MD, PhD and David L. Suskind, MD

A number of commercially available weight loss programs have previously targeted adults but are now targeting adolescents, youth, and even families. It is important as clinicians to acknowledge all choices that families have as they decide how to modify their lifestyles for improved health. Discussions about commercial weight loss programs can also set the stage for the health care provider to initiate a conversation regarding the best program for the particular child.[1]

Choice for an appropriate weight loss program should be individualized and based on the child's age, the severity of comorbidities, and body mass index. No one-size-fits-all program exists in the pediatric population. Preteens are actively growing and thus need higher protein, minerals, and vitamins in their diets. Restriction in these dietary components can have a significant negative impact on their overall growth. Similarly, the dietary needs of each child may differ because of child-dependent factors such as puberty and growth rate and physical activity levels (eg, sports activities). Additional program considerations include the emotional development of the child and the social and socioeconomic situation of the family.

Critical to a successful weight loss program is the institution of an effective, safe exercise program. Such programs emphasize the importance of changing the current energy balance in favor of expenditure over intake. In general, most programs encourage replacing sedentary with active, whole-body movement activities. However, before instituting an exercise program or regimen, the safety of that program needs to be ascertained (refer to Question 13).

Motivation to lose weight is the key essential factor both in losing and maintaining an ideal body weight. Motivation needs to come from within the individual/family and must be supported by the weight loss program. Reinforcement of prescribed changes in dietary patterns and physical activity is key to successful behavioral weight loss programs and should be scheduled regularly.

Huang JS, ed. *Curbside Consultation in Pediatric Obesity: 49 Clinical Questions* (pp 213-215).
© 2014 Taylor & Francis Group

Behavioral motivations from different weight management programs can be delivered via a variety of formats, including individual counseling, group workshops, and Internet programs.

One difficulty in discussing commercially available weight loss programs with families lies in the fact that most weight loss programs are primarily designed for adults. In addition, these programs have not generally been tested in children and thus lack evidence regarding their safety and efficacy in youth. Variations in the needs of the pediatric consumer and the sheer variety and volume of programs available add to the complexity. Nevertheless, in published research, some structured commercial weight loss programs have been shown to be superior to self-help and counseling in managing overweight adults.[2] However, results from adult studies can be extrapolated to children only to a certain degree. In addition, these studies are commonly performed by the programs themselves and are subject to bias. Furthermore, studies comparing major commercial weight loss programs head to head are scarce, thus making it hard for the health care provider to recommend one program over another.

The 4 main aspects of a commercial weight management program that are reported to the Federal Trade Commission (not the FDA) include the following: key components of the program, support staff qualifications, cost of the program, and potential risks of the treatment. A key component of any weight management program is administering a lowered-calorie diet either as pre-packaged meals or having the clients prepare the meals. All programs provide support in the forms of group or individual sessions aiming at behavioral modification. Enhancing physical activity is also a common focus for all, with some programs providing booklets, audio or video recordings, seminars, and member-made plans with their health care providers. Staff qualifications can range from licensed physicians (Health Management Resources, OPTIFAST), registered dieticians, company-trained counselors (Jenny Craig, LA Weight Loss, eDiets.com), or a leader elected at a local chapter (Overeaters Anonymous). This aspect of the program can change based on the success or failure of the program, with better revenue generation ideally leading to employment of licensed professionals, although not guaranteed. Costs of commercially available programs can range anywhere from hundreds to thousands of dollars over a span of a few months. Health Management Resources and OPTIFAST programs include medical visits and laboratory tests, which make these programs more expensive as compared with Overeaters Anonymous, which is virtually free for all. Although it is reasonable to consider these programs as safe, corresponding safety data are lacking. With regard to their efficacy, it is fair to assume that most programs are effective if all directions are followed per manufacturer's instructions. However, client adherence is unlikely to be 100% all of the time, and long-term efficacy data are not present.

Among all the commercial weight loss programs available, the Weight Watchers program has been evaluated in children aged older than 10 years and shown to be successful.[3] A partnership program between Tennessee Medicaid and Weight Watchers allowed recipients to attend the program at no out-of-pocket cost. Although this nonconcurrent prospective study has some limitations, it is one of the few studies in the pediatric population that provides evidence on the efficacy of a structured weight loss program. The majority of enrolled children with even minimal intervention were able to either meet or exceed the recommendations of the Expert Committee Recommendations Regarding the Prevention, Assessment, and Treatment of Childhood and Adolescent Overweight and Obesity.[4] This type of partnership can thus give low-income families an opportunity to participate in a program with a good chance of success at much less cost to the health care system.

Conclusion

No one-size-fits-all program exists in the world of weight management for children. Safety and efficacy for long-term maintenance are of paramount importance, but data are lacking for most commercially available weight loss programs for children. Nevertheless, recommending commercially available weight loss programs to children could work if chosen appropriately, keeping in mind the specific needs in the pediatric population for their growth and nutrition. Without question, the best approach to losing and maintaining an ideal body weight in children is helping influence the child and the world in which he or she lives, including parents who shape that world.

References

1. Tsai AG, Wadden TA. Systematic review: an evaluation of major commercial weight loss programs in the United States. *Ann Intern Med.* 2005;142(1):56-66.
2. Heshka S, Anderson JW, Atkinson RL, et al. Weight loss with self-help compared with a structured commercial program: a randomized trial. *JAMA.* 2003;289(14):1792-1798.
3. Mitchell NS, Suh CA, Stroebele N, Hill JO, Tsai AG. Weight change in pediatric TennCare recipients referred to a commercial weight loss program. *Acad Pediatr.* 2013;13(2):152-158.
4. Barlow SE; Expert Committee. Expert Committee recommendations regarding the prevention, assessment, and treatment of child and adolescent overweight and obesity: summary report. *Pediatrics.* 2007;120(Suppl 4): S164-S192.

SECTION VII

OTHER

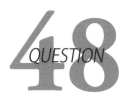

WHAT ARE THE HEALTH CARE AND ECONOMIC COSTS OF PEDIATRIC OBESITY?

Leonardo Trasande, MD, MPP and Tamasyn Nelson, DO

Obesity perhaps produces the largest increases in health care costs because of its association with multiple comorbidities, including asthma, sleep apnea, hyperlipidemia, glucose intolerance, hepatic steatosis, and cholelithiasis. With the advent of these formerly adult chronic medical issues arising in childhood, we may witness this current generation of children being the first in history to have a shorter lifespan than their parents. Care for these comorbidities also produces a financial burden through increased health care use.

Health care costs of comorbidities of childhood obesity are underrecognized largely because of underdiagnosis and under-documentation of this condition. In a nationally representative sample of outpatient clinic visits, obesity was rarely diagnosed (13% of all well-child visits for children with elevated body mass index), and diagnosis of obesity was reserved for those who were most severely or obviously obese.[1] In a nationally representative sample of US hospitalizations, only 2% carried a secondary diagnosis of obesity, yet these few hospitalizations cost $237.6 million.[2] Although this is likely an underestimate, childhood obesity produces a large economic burden on society.

Compared with their normal-weight counterparts, overweight and obese children also have more outpatient and emergency room visits as well as hospitalizations. Evidence suggests that these direct costs of obesity are seen as early as age 6 years. In a study of health care costs of obese and overweight 6- to 19-year-old patients, the cost of health care for these children and adolescents was estimated to be an additional $2.9 billion annually, due to increased use of prescription drugs, outpatient visits, and visits to the emergency room.[3] There are other social costs unrelated to medical care that are direct consequences of childhood obesity. Children who are obese are more likely to suffer from psychosocial stress and miss more school. This absenteeism may indirectly reduce economic productivity in later life.

Huang JS, ed. *Curbside Consultation in Pediatric Obesity: 49 Clinical Questions* (pp 219-220).
© 2014 Taylor & Francis Group

Perhaps the largest social cost is the lost quality of life of these obese and overweight children over a lifetime. Studies have quantified this lost quality of life using quality-adjusted life years, which are measures of the perceptions of quality of life as compared in those with disease and those with perfect health. For example, in comparison between a patient in perfect health and a diabetic person, for a given year the diabetic patient may report a 20% decreased perceived quality of life due to increased doctor visits, medication use, etc. A study published in 2010 suggests that compared with a patient in perfect health, an obese person may report a 5% decreased perceived quality of life with respect to morbidity and mortality.[4] Typically society values quality-adjusted life years in the range of $50,000 each, and so potentially large social costs can be produced from childhood obesity.

Economic principles and interventions can help us understand the economic causes of obesity. From a policy standpoint, it can also allow us to compare various existing interventions on the same terms. For example, changes in agricultural policy could positively affect availability of healthier food options that may lead to a reduction in childhood obesity. This would require a shift from the current policies that subsidize calorically dense crops, such as corn, to providing policy incentives to produce alternate healthier crops[5,6] that are not as calorically dense, such as fruits, which would enable families to make healthier and economically sound decisions for food choices.

Because of the difficulty in treating established obesity and the impact it has on economic factors and social factors for the individual as well as for society, effective preventive strategies and interventions are urgently needed. However, given the relative ineffectiveness of individual-level interventions to prevent obesity in childhood to date, policy makers are now considering larger changes in environmental factors that also contribute to obesity in childhood.

Preventing childhood obesity and overweight will require a broad approach. Additional research to identify preventable risk factors such as educational interventions in schools, homes, and other settings, including improvements in nutrition labeling, new guidelines for marketing foods to youth, and changes in the "built environment," will be needed. A recent study has shown that spending 2 billion dollars a year for the 12-year-old cohort could be cost effective when the interventions funded are successful in reducing the prevalence of childhood obesity by just 1%.[7] These results suggest that additional research into interventions is necessary and that even some costly interventions of uncertain efficacy may be worth pursuing.

Pediatricians and general practitioners are poised to be effective advocates in raising policy maker awareness of the negative health effects and increasing costs associated with childhood obesity. They can also educate policy makers about the need for broader environmental interventions to combat the epidemic, given that behavioral change can be difficult to accomplish and maintain.

References

1. Hampl SE, Carroll CA, Simon SD, Sharma V. Resource utilization and expenditures for overweight and obese children. *JAMA Pediatrics*. 2007;161(1):11-14.
2. Trasande L, Liu Y, Fryer G, Weitzman M. Effects of childhood obesity on hospital care and costs, 1999-2005. *Health Aff (Millwood)*. 2009;28(4):w751-w760.
3. Trasande L, Chatterjee S. The impact of obesity on health service utilization and costs in childhood. *Obesity (Silver Spring)*. 2009;17(9):1749-1754.
4. Jia H, Lubetkin E. Obesity-related quality-adjusted life years lost in the U.S. from 1993 to 2008. *Am J Prev Med*. 2010;39(3):220-227.
5. Cawley J. The economics of childhood obesity. *Health Aff (Milwood)*. 2010;29(3):364-371.
6. Wallinga D. Agricultural policy and childhood obesity: a food systems and public health commentary. *Health Aff (Milwood)*. 2010;29(3):372-378.
7. Trasande L. How much should we invest in preventing childhood obesity? *Health Aff (Milwood)*. 2010;29(3):372-378.

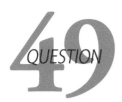

HOW SHOULD PHYSICIANS
ADVOCATE FOR PEDIATRIC OBESITY?
HOW DOES ONE GET STARTED?

Christine Wood, MD, FAAP, CLE

Giving advice to a family with an overweight or obese child can be fraught with frustration, which is understandable considering that the advice we give families may turn out to be unrealistic because of barriers in their environment and in their community. Even if families know the healthy food choices, it might be difficult for them to make those choices. For example, if we tell families to increase their fruit and vegetable intake but their neighborhoods have no full-service grocery stores, a limited availability of fruits and vegetables, and a high density of fast food restaurants, finding fruits and vegetables becomes a challenge. Similarly, if we recommend more physical activity but their neighborhood has parks overtaken by the homeless or gangs, or there is a lack of safe walking or biking paths, getting more physical activity becomes difficult.

Advocacy is a way for physicians to go beyond the 4 walls of their practice. The impact of being a pediatric obesity advocate in your community can promote solutions that can be broader and far reaching. If we look at the dictionary definition of the word *advocacy*, it means: speaking out, expressing one's opinion on a matter of importance; the act of supporting a cause or proposal; storytelling; and leadership. All of these definitions are important in being a pediatric obesity advocate. The public respects your opinion, and by leveraging your medical expertise and using your credibility, you can become an effective messenger on obesity-prevention issues. In taking your first steps in advocacy, understand that there are different levels of time commitment and depth of involvement, but even a few small advocacy projects performed by many different people can make a large impact on a community. Also, by finding community partners already doing work in this area, you can build on existing efforts and may not need to start from the ground up.

The following are some first step items to consider in becoming a pediatric obesity advocate.

1. **Understand the Problem.** Pediatric obesity is in the news, so stay up-to-date on the topic. Sign up for news feeds and read resources from organizations that deal with policy (see

Huang JS, ed. *Curbside Consultation in
Pediatric Obesity: 49 Clinical Questions* (pp 221-223).
© 2014 Taylor & Francis Group

Suggested Readings) and scour your pediatric journals for articles that address the pediatric obesity issue. A number of excellent policy statements from the American Academy of Pediatrics (AAP) engage community topics, like "The Crucial Role of Recess in School"[1] and "The Built Environment: Designing Communities to Promote Physical Activity in Children."[2] These help give a perspective on how the AAP approaches the role of pediatricians in environmental change to increase physical activity in children.

Sharing real stories from your practice and from your community is a powerful part of telling your story as you do your advocacy work. They say that facts tell and stories sell, and so real-life examples are important to incorporate. Borrowing examples and stories from other communities is also acceptable. To set an agenda for your work, you may then want to pick a specific topic that you can become passionate about, like reducing sugar-sweetened beverages; this could then lead to work in preschools, schools, hospitals, or medical offices, and other venues to bring your goal to fruition.

2. **Find Local Partners.** As practicing pediatricians, we know the schools and preschools in our communities. Contact them and see if they would like a guest speaker on nutrition or an article written for their parents and staff. Find out what type of school wellness policy they have or if there is a wellness committee at the local school, and volunteer to be part of that committee. If you have your own children, it is even easier to get involved because you probably have a vested interest in how your own child's environment is structured, so talk to your child's preschool, school, sports team, or place of worship and offer your expertise. Remember, it is important to have school officials see your role as a voice to add value to the organization and not as a critic about what the organization is doing wrong. Offer solutions, not complaints.

3. **Find Broader Partners.** On a larger scale, find other coalitions or organizations that are already conducting obesity advocacy work in your community. If you contact these groups, they will often be eager and receptive to having a medical expert to work with, so don't be shy about inquiring. This may include your local health department, local hospitals, or youth groups (eg, YMCA, Boys and Girls Clubs). Of course, there are even broader ways to get involved with local government, elected officials, or national organizations. A simple e-mail message to an organization or key decision maker may be a way to open doors to your advocacy journey.

4. **Tailor Your Message.** Different audiences will need different messages. When talking to parents, offer simple, practical solutions and resources. Help them feel like you are on their side and empathize with their challenges. Avoid lecturing parents about things they are doing wrong and try to offer solutions that are realistic and within reach. I often tell families that it is not about achieving perfection and making sudden changes in what we do, but rather about gradually making small changes in nutrition and lifestyle to make progress toward new habits. When talking to staff who work with children, like teachers, administrators, coaches, or even the general public, explain the impact of childhood obesity to society and how change can create benefits for their organization or for society in general. Having examples of broader-reaching policies in organizations similar to their own can offer inspiration that change is possible. If you are dealing with high-level policy makers, such as elected officials or large organizations, an overview with facts that address their own constituency or organization can be powerful. Follow up by then making the case for how policy within their constituency or organization can make an impact on health, productivity, finances or absences because of health.

5. **Method of Communication.** You need to decide how you want to share your message. Offering to write an article for a school newsletter, local paper, or local parenting magazine may be an easy place to start. Offering your services as a speaker is usually appreciated by

parents who want more information about healthy lifestyles for their children. Of course, larger audiences can be reached with television or larger circulation newspapers. And finally, if you are collaborating with community partners from other sectors working on childhood obesity, your method of communication may be by attending meetings and supporting ongoing efforts and offering your expertise.

An example of how advocacy can work with physician involvement is the collaborative model from San Diego, California: the San Diego County Childhood Obesity Initiative (COI). This was founded in 2006 as a public/private partnership whose mission is to reduce and prevent childhood obesity in San Diego County by creating healthy environments for all children and families through advocacy, education, policy development, and environmental change. The COI engages community partners from multiple sectors to work together to affect childhood obesity and works in 7 domains, including government, health care, schools, early childhood, community, media, and business. Specifically, the work within the COI health care domain involves individual health providers, including pediatricians, family practice, psychiatrists, obstetricians, and school nurses; women, infants, and children (WIC) staff and dietitians; and partners from local hospitals, the San Diego County Medical Society, and the local AAP chapter. One recent collaborative project involved training offered by a pediatric physician advocate and a WIC staff representative to provide a lunchtime training to primary care offices about WIC services, nutrition, activity messages, and updated food packages. Pre- and post-surveys found that the office staff and physicians learned new information about WIC that they did not know and thus were able to make better use of the WIC services after the training. Another project that is being explored is the Nutrition in Healthcare Leadership Team, in which several major local hospitals will meet to collaborate on healthy food procurement and a hospital-wide Rethink Your Drink campaign that has been successfully launched at Rady Children's Hospital.

San Diego is fortunate to have a working, established model with the San Diego County Childhood Obesity Initiative, but physicians in all communities can find ways to get involved on a large or small scale. If everyone could put in 20 hours a year in advocacy, thousands of hours of work could be accomplished in our communities. Our vision in medicine is to support the wellness of our patients, but supporting the wellness of our communities is a crucial and equally important part of the puzzle to solve our childhood obesity crisis.

References

1. Murray R, Ramstetter C; Council on School Health; American Academy of Pediatrics. The crucial role of recess in school. *Pediatrics*. 2013;131(1);183-188.
2. Committee on Environmental Health, Tester JM. The built environment: designing communities to promote physical activity in children. *Pediatrics*. 2009;123(6):1591-1598.

Suggested Readings

American Academy of Pediatrics. Prevention and Treatment of Childhood Overweight and Obesity: Policy Opportunities Tool. http://www2.aap.org/obesity/matrix_1.html. Accessed November 6, 2013.

California Medical Association Foundation. Obesity Prevention Project. http://www.thecmafoundation.org/projects/obesityProject.aspx. Accessed November 6, 2013.

National Initiative for Children's Healthcare Quality. Be Our Voice. http://www.nichq.org/advocacy. Accessed November 6, 2013.

Robert Wood Johnson Foundation. http://www.rwjf.org (search topic of childhood obesity). Accessed November 6, 2013.

San Diego County Childhood Obesity Initiative. http://www.ourcommunityourkids.org. Accessed November 6, 2013.

FINANCIAL DISCLOSURES

Dr. Richard L. Atkinson is the owner of Obetech, LLC. Obetech provides assays for adenoviruses that produce obesity and has several patents in the area of virus-induced obesity, including for diagnostic assays, antiviral agents, and vaccines.

Dr. Frank M. Biro has no financial or proprietary interest in the materials presented herein.

Dr. Christopher F. Bolling has no financial or proprietary interest in the materials presented herein.

Dr. Kerri N. Boutelle has no financial or proprietary interest in the materials presented herein.

Dr. Abby L. Braden has no financial or proprietary interest in the materials presented herein.

Dr. Lillian J. Choi has no financial or proprietary interest in the materials presented herein.

Dr. Alison M. Coates has no financial or proprietary interest in the materials presented herein.

Dr. Lee Ann E. Conard has no financial or proprietary interest in the materials presented herein.

Dr. Ellen L. Connor has no financial or proprietary interest in the materials presented herein.

Dr. Brian Dauenhauer has no financial or proprietary interest in the materials presented herein.

Dr. Christopher Davis has no financial or proprietary interest in the materials presented herein.

Angela Estampador has no financial or proprietary interest in the materials presented herein.

Dr. Katherine M. Flegal has no financial or proprietary interest in the materials presented herein.

Dr. Andrei Fodoreanu has no financial or proprietary interest in the materials presented herein.

Dr. Paul W. Franks has no financial or proprietary interest in the materials presented herein.

Jeanette M. Garcia has no financial or proprietary interest in the materials presented herein.

Dr. Mary Abigail S. Garcia has no financial or proprietary interest in the materials presented herein.

Dara Garner-Edwards has no financial or proprietary interest in the materials presented herein.

Dr. Michael Gottschalk is a consultant for Daiichi Sankyo and receives research funding from Eli Lily and Versartis.

Dr. David Gozal has no financial or proprietary interest in the materials presented herein.

Dr. H. Mollie Grow has no financial or proprietary interest in the materials presented herein.

Dr. Rohit Gupta has no financial or proprietary interest in the materials presented herein.

Dr. Sarah Hampl has no financial or proprietary interest in the materials presented herein.

Dr. Sandra Hassink has no financial or proprietary interest in the materials presented herein.

Dr. Kimberly Henrichs has no financial or proprietary interest in the materials presented herein.

Dr. Krista Beth Highland has no financial or proprietary interest in the materials presented herein.

Dr. Linda L. Hill has no financial or proprietary interest in the materials presented herein.

Dr. Stefanie N. Hinkle has no financial or proprietary interest in the materials presented herein.

Dr. Nancy Hoo has no financial or proprietary interest in the materials presented herein.

Dr. Jeannie S. Huang has no financial or proprietary interest in the materials presented herein.

Dr. Sherry Huang has no financial or proprietary interest in the materials presented herein.

Dr. Xiaofen Deng Keating has no financial or proprietary interest in the materials presented herein.

Dr. Jacqueline Kerr has no financial or proprietary interest in the materials presented herein.

Dr. Brian K. Kit has no financial or proprietary interest in the materials presented herein.

Dr. Stephanie Knatz has no financial or proprietary interest in the materials presented herein.

Dr. Heather M. Kong has no financial or proprietary interest in the materials presented herein.

Dr. Kirsten La has no financial or proprietary interest in the materials presented herein.

Dr. Jennifer Le has no financial or proprietary interest in the materials presented herein.

Dr. Colleen Taylor Lukens has no financial or proprietary interest in the materials presented herein.

Dr. Kimberly Montez has no financial or proprietary interest in the materials presented herein.

Dr. Tamasyn Nelson has no financial or proprietary interest in the materials presented herein.

Dr. Kimberly P. Newton has no financial or proprietary interest in the materials presented herein.

Dr. Kevin Patrick is co-founder of Santech, Inc.

Dr. Denise Purdie has no financial or proprietary interest in the materials presented herein.

Dr. Kyung E. Rhee has no financial or proprietary interest in the materials presented herein.

Dr. Sanjeev Sabharwal has no financial or proprietary interest in the materials presented herein.

Dr. Jeffrey B. Schwimmer has no financial or proprietary interest in the materials presented herein.

Dr. Rulan Shangguan has no financial or proprietary interest in the materials presented herein.

Dr. Andrea J. Sharma has no financial or proprietary interest in the materials presented herein.

Dr. John R. Sirard has no financial or proprietary interest in the materials presented herein.

Dr. Joseph A. Skelton has no financial or proprietary interest in the materials presented herein.

Karen Stephens has no financial or proprietary interest in the materials presented herein.

Dr. David L. Suskind has no financial or proprietary interest in the materials presented herein.

Dr. Kenneth P. Tercyak has no financial or proprietary interest in the materials presented herein.

Dr. Leonardo Trasande has no financial or proprietary interest in the materials presented herein.

Dr. Patrika Tsai has no financial or proprietary interest in the materials presented herein.

Dr. Raymond J. Tseng has no financial or proprietary interest in the materials presented herein.

Dr. Margarita D. Tsiros has no financial or proprietary interest in the materials presented herein.

Dr. Victor E. Uko has no financial or proprietary interest in the materials presented herein.

Dr. Christine Wood has no financial or proprietary interest in the materials presented herein.

Dr. Stravra A. Xanthakos has no financial or proprietary interest in the materials presented herein.

INDEX

Printed in the United States
by Baker & Taylor Publisher Services